GET FIT AND HEALTHY ON A TIGHT SCHEDULE
2 BOOKS IN 1

By Silvana Siskov

GET FIT AND HEALTHY ON A TIGHT SCHEDULE 2 BOOKS IN 1
LIVE HEALTHY ON A TIGHT SCHEDULE
GET FIT AND HEALTHY IN YOUR OWN HOME IN 20 MINUTES OR LESS
www.silvanasiskov.com

Copyright © 2020 SILVANA SISKOV

PAPERBACK ISBN: 978-1-9162424-6-3

Limits of Liability and Disclaimer of Warranty

The author and publisher shall not be liable for your misuse of the enclosed material. This book is strictly for informational and educational purposes only.

Warning Disclaimer

The purpose of this book is to educate and entertain. The author and/or publisher do not guarantee that anyone following these techniques, suggestions, tips, ideas, or strategies will become successful. The author and/or publisher shall have neither liability nor responsibility to anyone with respect to any loss or damage caused, or alleged to be caused, directly or indirectly by the information contained in this book.

Medical Disclaimer

The medical or health information in this book is provided as an information resource only, and is not to be used or relied on for any diagnostic or treatment purposes. This information is not intended to be patient education, does not create any patient-physician relationship, and should not be used as a substitute for professional diagnosis and treatment.

Printed in the United States and the United Kingdom.

Table of Contents

BOOK 2

GET FIT AND HEALTHY IN YOUR OWN HOME IN 20 MINUTES OR LESS

LIVE HEALTHY ON A TIGHT SCHEDULE

5 Easy Ways for Busy People to Develop Sustainable Habits Around Food, Exercise and Self-Care

By Silvana Siskov

Thank you for purchasing
Live Healthy on a Tight Schedule:
5 Easy Ways for Busy People to Develop Sustainable
Habits Around Food, Exercise and Self-Care

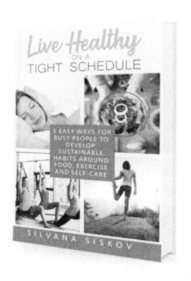

As a special thank you for purchasing this book,
go to www.bit.ly/bundle-fit-and-healthy
and download your
"5 Day Healthy Meal Plan for Busy People."
You will also receive a special bonus:
"20 Items That You Must Have on Your Food
Shopping List."

Go to www.bit.ly/bundle-fit-and-healthy.

Dear Reader

Are you finding life too busy, and you are juggling many things at the same time?

Are you struggling to find time to prepare healthy meals?

Are you finding it challenging to make time to exercise?

Are you struggling to find time for self-care?

Are you wondering how to have a healthy lifestyle whilst living life on a tight schedule?

If this is how you feel, believe me, you are not alone. I have spent many years working with clients of different ages, genders, and professions, and I keep noticing, over and over again, that eating properly, exercising regularly, going to bed earlier, and focusing on self-care, are the things that most people want to achieve, but they do not know how.

I can also see that dealing with stress and pressure, and coping with demands of everyday life, are common problems in today's society. They limit our ability, affect willpower, and take away our motivation to be the best we can be.

Many studies have been done over the last few years, and researchers are finding increased evidence towards modern life's negative effect on our physical and mental health. More and more people are experiencing ill health, and a large population of people is struggling to find the answers and solutions to their unhealthy daily routines.

Many individuals experience high levels of stress and suffer from anxiety and depression. The need for consuming stimulants such as caffeine and sugary snacks, which only temporarily help with the increase of energy levels, is on the rise. Obesity is on the rise too, and the number of people receiving a diagnosis of cardiovascular disease and type 2 diabetes is growing. It is truly worrying to see that so many deaths are caused by diseases that are easily preventable.

The purpose of this book is to show you how developing new and healthy habits can enhance your life, whilst getting rid of old and unhealthy habits that are damaging to your health. Creating healthy habits is not too hard, even when you are a busy person.

It is important to understand that whatever you want to achieve, whether you want to be healthier, live longer, be a successful athlete, have a successful business, lose weight, or anything else, the main principles driving you towards your goals are always the same. The outline of the process that you need to follow is exactly the same: You must know what your goal is and why you want it. You need to have a clear vision in your mind, and you have to be willing to commit to your success.

This is how these principles work in practice:

Principle 1: Know Your "Why"

Your "why" is the vehicle to your destination. It creates desire to move you forward and gives you the strength to take you towards your goal, even at times when you are struggling or feeling depleted.

Knowing why you do what you do creates purpose and gives meaning to your actions. Your "why" will always show you the way, despite your environment and the circumstances you live in. If you are unsure about your reasons why you must change your behaviour, and how this change can impact your life, your motivation will soon desert you, and you will not achieve your desired goal.

It is very easy to say, "I want to eat healthy and exercise a few times a week," but unless you know why you want it, and how you will benefit from it, you will struggle to achieve your goal.

Principle 2: Have a Clear Vision

You can achieve nearly anything you want in life, but to do this, it is necessary to create a clear vision and be clear about your goals. Without knowing your exact goals, you will not know where you are going, or which path to follow in order to get there.

It is simple: Be specific about what you want. When thinking about your future, make sure you can see a broad picture in your mind. This will provide you with clarity, ambition, and energy. It will make you feel enthusiastic when talking about your future goals and excited when working towards them. It will provide you with the desire and motivation, even at times when you feel tired and frail. It will give you a push and inspire your actions, so working towards your goals will become a strong desire, rather than a chore with no purpose and fulfilment.

Knowing what you want to achieve and why you want it is the best motivation that you can get in life. Nothing can be as motivating and inspiring as working towards something that you want and knowing that your efforts and energy will be rewarded in the end.

Principle 3: Commit to Your Success

To achieve what you want, I suggest that you start from the end and work towards the beginning; you are effectively working backwards! Knowing your "why," and having a clear vision, will help you with this process and combined together, they create commitment.

Any journey has the beginning, the middle, and the end. The beginning is the place where your motivation is high. This is the place where your dreams are born and plans for the future start taking shape. The middle part is where your commitment supports your actions at times when you struggle the most. The end is your future. This is where your goals are accomplished and your dreams come to life.

Visualise your success and where you want to be, then follow the path that takes you there. You will probably face many challenges and barriers on the way, but the commitment to achieve your goal has to be stronger than your wish to live without it. Put simply, you have to want it with everything you have.

Your hunger and desire to achieve what you want are impacted by the degree of your motivation, but let me tell you something: Without commitment, you will struggle and will not succeed when your motivation fades, which it will at some point. Your ability to get what you want is not only affected by how much you really want it, but how hard you work for it too.

These principles play an important role in determining your success in achieving your goals.

Following the steps in this book will lead you towards reaching your goals — whether it is to feel less stressed, be slimmer, or to feel healthier — whatever it is that you desire for yourself.

Focus on one step at a time, and work on it until it becomes a habit.

However, it is important to realise that whilst going through life, you will be required to make many changes and to adjust your behaviours many times over, according to the circumstances at the time. Try not to be discouraged by this and lose faith in your own abilities when things get tough. Remember, you are in control of your reactions, and you are the leader of your actions towards anything that life throws at you.

You are the author of your life.

Chapter 1: Habits

"We first make our habits, then our habits make us."

John Dryden

How to Develop Healthy Habits

First things first, it is important to understand the power of habits. You can easily use your own habits for good or bad, but identifying your own personal habits and changing them towards the positive end of the scale will serve you well as a firm foundation on which to build your healthier lifestyle from scratch.

Developing healthy habits forms a cornerstone to a healthy life, and the impact they have on our health and well-being is crucial. You cannot live a healthy life if you continue to indulge in habits that are to the detriment of your health and well-being. If you constantly overeat when you feel emotional, you are going to sabotage any efforts towards losing weight. If you always procrastinate when you are feeling under a little pressure, you are going to put off the things that are important and never achieve what you really want to achieve.

Habits are both good and bad, but you can control them for yourself and use them for your greater good.

One of the things that most of us wish for ourselves is to be healthy. Health is the most important thing you can have in life. Many people believe that being healthy, slim, and fit, is hard to achieve. Actually, focusing on health in general is far easier than most people think. However, for this to happen, for you to actually become healthier, you need to realise that changes need to be made. You need to make decisions to change your diet, lose weight, or start an exercise regime. However, motivation is often short-lived, and learning to extend it is key.

A healthy lifestyle requires you to develop long-term healthy habits, and this is something that most people usually struggle with, simply because they do not know where to start. This struggle often contributes to the loss of motivation, and when motivation is gone, disappointment quickly takes over. Feeling this way tends to pull us back to our old habits and behaviours, with a dose of self-loathing as a result of the perceived failure.

Of course, not achieving something is not necessarily a failure, but allowing your motivation to desert you, and not doing anything about getting it back, is something that needs to be addressed.

Understanding that your new habits cannot be developed overnight is vital. It takes time to create them, and it takes energy to practise them. Only after many regular repetitions can they become a part of your regular behavioural pattern. However, creating healthy habits does not need to be hard work, and it is often simply a matter of adding a new pattern of behaviour to your existing, well-established behaviour. This is a very simple way of managing your well-being, although no one can deny that it takes time and effort.

If you carry on doing what you have always done, you will get what you always had. It is that simple. Finding excuses for being too busy, and putting blame on others for the inability to have the life you want, will not bring you success. Developing new and healthy habits can only start, and be maintained, by having determination to succeed, and understanding how your new behaviour can change your life. It is not about relying on other people or circumstances, but creating the circumstances that you want to live in. You have the control in your own hands, and you need to open your heart and your eyes to the fact that the only person who can sabotage your efforts is you, and the only person who can help you onwards, is also you.

To achieve what you want, whatever it is, you have to start with creating new habits. The best way to achieve this is to add a new behaviour to your existing habits, and soon afterwards you will notice that your new behaviour is turning into a new habit, by replacing the old behavioural pattern. How to follow this part of the process will be discussed later on in this book, but for now, simply be mindful of the fact that old habits can be changed, and new ones can be added.

We all have habits, and they help us get through life. However, a habit is more than just something we do often. There is normally a trigger that starts the action, and a pay-off that gives us pleasure. The problem comes when it is a short-term pleasure that is bad for us in the long run. For example, the trigger for eating something unhealthy may be anything from feeling depressed or bored to passing a vending machine. The pay-off is the short-term high that sugary or fatty food can give, but that is soon replaced by a low, when you realise you are putting on weight and do not have the energy you need.

One of the major problems in developing healthy habits is that the pay-off is usually more immediate and obvious for unhealthy habits. For instance, an immediate sugar rush from unhealthy food as opposed to the long-term benefits of healthy eating. Or lounging on the sofa, watching your favourite TV programme, rather than going out for a run in the middle of a winter's day, when the weather is cold and it is dark outside.

This is the reason why it is vital to be clear about the benefits of your healthy habits. When you know why something is going to benefit you, it is easier to stay focused upon achieving it as a goal. Understanding the benefits of making any sort of change in life can help you to overcome the lure of unhealthy, but instant, gratification.

The effect of your habits on your everyday life is enormous, and should never be underestimated. Most of your behaviours are determined by the long-term habits you have repeated a number of times before, and as such, they have become your way of life.

Some habits are good and others are bad, but all of them are equally important as they create the foundation on which your daily routines are built. The routines that you develop affect all areas of your life, and play a significant role in your health, finances, relationships, etc. The key is to determine which habits are damaging to you and which ones benefit you. By doing that, you can change the damaging ones and increase your focus on the beneficial ones.

Most of the habits you currently have were developed a long time ago. They have been formed through consistency and repetition, to the point where you probably do not even realise you are doing them. That is the reason why, even when the habits are not doing you any favours, you make excuses for their existence in order to protect them. You feel loyal to them, and you find it hard to let them go. They are part and parcel of your life and who you are to a large degree.

I understand this. Let's be honest; you have spent months, years, and even decades in their company. You have been living with them, sleeping with them, and then they became your family and your best friend. It is hard to imagine living your life without them, and when you start to try and change them, it is normal to feel a little nervous or even slightly lost. The good news is, this will pass.

Of course, I agree that creating new and healthy habits, and getting rid of your old and unhealthy habits, is not always easy when life is so busy and terribly stressful. But, focusing on what really matters to you will help you develop a different type of mindset, and it is this mindset that will allow you to overcome challenges in your new healthier lifestyle plan.

Your new mindset will also support you in creating new patterns of behaviour and provide you with an opportunity to make your body healthier, working towards a more fulfilling life. Feeling good about yourself will encourage you to embrace the change, and as a result you will notice your confidence beginning to soar. When that happens, anything is possible.

It is important to remember that the aim of establishing healthy habits is not to restrict yourself but to enhance your life beyond what it is right now. This is a life built on healthy habits, containing all the great ingredients required for health and happiness, including healthy thoughts, healthy attitude, healthy words, and healthy actions. Becoming healthier is not all about eating more fruits and vegetables and moving your body more; it is about loving who you are and making time for yourself too. It is an entire package deal that needs to be embraced fully if you want the effects to snowball into something that makes a real difference in your life.

I would like to remind you that the perfect start for creating a healthy habit that leads towards a new behaviour is to visualise where you want to be and why. Visualise your end point. Let your vision be your guide. Imagine the end result, and work towards the beginning. By doing this, you will subconsciously create a path in your mind that will take you to your goal. It might seem like you are working backwards in many ways, but you are already motivated by this point because you have seen what it will look like and feel like if you achieve it. That is the ultimate motivation.

If your goal is to have less stress and more relaxation, less anxiety and more calmness, less illness and more health, less worry and more joy, then your action plan must include creating a lifestyle that will prioritise things that can give you relaxation, calmness, health, and joy. This includes developing healthy lifestyle habits, healthy eating habits, a healthy relationship with yourself and others, and understanding your own needs.

Making only one small step at a time is enough. Often, it is more than enough. Each step will move you forward and bring your goals closer to you.

Now, imagine if you decided to make just one small change in your behaviour every day of the week. That would be 365 changed habits this time next year. Would your life be different in any way if you did this? What do you think?

Okay, maybe changing your behaviour every day sounds too overwhelming. If this is the case, then focus on making one small change in your behaviour once per week. That will be 52 changes in your behaviour this time next year. Do you think that making 52 changes in your behaviour, and creating 52 new habits, will improve your life? Of course, it will.

Can you think of the ways in which your life could improve by doing this? I am sure you can think of many, and those changes will turn into even bigger benefits the more energy you focus towards them.

The most important aspect about your habits is to remember that they are not fixed. All your habits were created because they served the purpose at the time. Every single habit you have right now, was consciously created, unconsciously accepted, and it became a part of your life because you carried on doing it. You can change your unwanted habits that work against you, and swap them with those that work for you.

In addition, you can change them any time you wish and any way you like, but in order for you to benefit from them, you need to make sure that your new habits fit your life, accommodate your needs, and take you towards the path that leads towards your goal.

Another thing to remember is that when it comes to creating a new habit, you need to make your new behaviour your point of focus. Stop searching for excuses that could prevent you from doing your best.

I know that working on developing a new habit, which eventually becomes your standard behaviour often seems like a difficult task to do. And it is especially hard when you are at the initial stage of creating a change. But focusing on your new behaviour has to be on the top of your priority list, and it has to stay there until it becomes a habit, despite the difficulties you might be experiencing on the way. Your efforts will pay off in the end, when you notice that your new habits are responsible for bringing many positive changes in your life.

Ultimately, I would like you to remember that you are in control of your behaviour. You are in control of all your actions. It is only you who can make the change, and any change that you make will eventually create a big difference in your life, the way you feel, and of course, to your future too.

How to Develop a Healthy Lifestyle

Most people believe that a healthy lifestyle includes only two things: a healthy diet and exercise. This is far from the truth.

A healthy lifestyle includes more than just eating healthy and exercising. It is about engaging with life in a way that is beneficial to the mind and body. This will help you create the balance between different areas of your life, and influence choices that you make on an everyday basis. Your mindset is the foundation towards a better life, and the stronger and more positive this is, the more chance you have of achieving exactly what you want and need.

There are many areas in life that often suffer because of a busy lifestyle. Later on in this book I will give you tips and guidance on diet and exercise, as well as the areas of your life that are often most neglected. Those areas include sleep and self-care. These are extremely important for our well-being, but they often suffer the most. By realising that health and well-being is a complete book of chapters and not just one small subject, you can ensure that you are ticking all the right boxes, and not missing important pieces of information.

As I discussed earlier, habits are made from the sets of behaviours that have been repeated time after time. All behaviours have triggers. In order to avoid your current unhealthy habits being triggered, it is important to understand what those triggers are, and develop strategies to help you avoid them. Whilst it might take a little soul searching to identify your true triggers, some are probably quite obvious too.

Of course, it can also be simple, such as planning your route so you do not pass the vending machine, or not having unhealthy food items in your fridge. On the other hand, if being lonely triggers comfort eating, you will need to find an alternative strategy to deal with it. By doing this, however, you are overcoming unhealthy habits that cause you to feel bad about yourself too, whilst also ensuring that you are ticking the healthy eating boxes at the same time.

As you can see, it is an open book, full of chapters that will benefit you in a myriad of ways.

It is also vital that you enjoy your healthy habits, as this will help you to avoid the temptation to slide back. This includes finding healthy foods you love eating, finding activities you love doing, and finding people you like spending time with.

This is crucial if you want to maintain your new approach over the long term.

In order to create healthy habits and develop healthy behaviours around diet, exercise, sleep, and self-care, it is important to focus on the tools that will benefit your life as opposed to damaging it. They include the following:

- Knowing your triggers
- Developing the right mindset
- Establishing a good relationship with your new habits
- Creating healthy daily routines
- Creating the environment that works for you

To help you develop a healthy lifestyle, it is important to create these five aspects, and they are all equally important. Let's explore their importance and talk about what you can do to make them happen, one by one.

Knowing Your Triggers

Understanding the reasons why you behave in a certain way, and the reasons you react to the triggers, will help you become more aware of your actions and your patterns of behaviour. My advice is to start paying attention to your triggers and the behaviours you display around them. You could even start a journal to help you understand more about your triggers and your behaviour when you encounter them.

Keep your diary for around two weeks or so, as anything less will not give you the right amount of information you need.

Then, after the time is finished, read back over your experiences during that time, and see if you can identify any patterns that might lead you towards identifying a trigger. Remember to write as much information as you can, as this will allow you to benefit from the journaling idea more.

Within this, remember to look for the external stimuli that are causing you to feel or behave a certain way, and identify your emotional response to it. I also advise you to look inside, evaluating your internal struggles and finding their cause. Awareness often creates an understanding, and this builds strength, helping us to create a shift in mindset. In addition, you will find better ways to handle perhaps emotional problems, which might cause you to act in a damaging way.

Developing the Right Mindset

I am sure you often hear the word *mindset*, but what is mindset?

The definition of the word *mindset* in the dictionary, is "a person's way of thinking and their opinions."

What this means in the context of this book is that you need to create a way of thinking that believes in the connection between good health and a healthy lifestyle. Only then will you be able to develop a love for healthy eating and commit to doing regular exercise and other activities that promote health. You also need to develop a healthy bedtime routine and find ways to reduce your stress levels.

If your mindset does not believe in healthy living, and refuses to adopt healthy lifestyle practises as part of your everyday life, you will then have a slim chance of succeeding. Of course, changing your mindset takes time and is not going to happen overnight; do not be discouraged if you do not see changes immediately, and instead stick with it and realise that the work you are doing is helping you move towards a healthier lifestyle overall. You will get there in the end.

Establishing a Good Relationship With Your New Habits

Once you have developed new habits, you need to enjoy them and learn to embrace them for all the good they are doing. Living healthy means you agree to do the following:

- Eat healthy and nutritious foods – This includes learning new and healthy recipes and experimenting with different ingredients that you might have never tried before.
- Do physical activities – Develop a love of fitness and get into the habit of moving your body a little more. You can do this by finding a sport or exercise you enjoy, or simply making it your aim to move your body a little more every single day.
- Quit or reduce using stimulants – This includes avoiding alcohol, tobacco, coffee, or sugary foods/drinks. Cutting stimulants such as these out of your life will benefit your health greatly, and will also give you more natural energy, as opposed to "fake" energy, which is likely to lead to a sugar crash later on.
- Make self-care your top priority – Learn how to reduce some of the stresses in your life, and focus on self-care as a top priority. Most people put off looking after

themselves, assuming that being there for others is more important. However, if you are not looking after yourself, how can you really be there for other people too?

These are the main factors that need attention when working towards a healthy lifestyle. The food you eat, the exercise you do, and the activities you practise around your own self-care are important elements in your daily life that you must not ignore. Learning to build healthy habits around these areas is crucial, as it will help you connect to your goal and your vision of living a healthy life. As a result, you will find it easier to achieve, with a stronger will to make these changes last.

In addition, I would like to encourage you to treat each relationship in your life equally. If you want to have a fit body, then you must not search for excuses when it comes to exercising. You must nurture your relationship with exercise, the same way as all other relationships that are important to you. If your goal is to live a long and healthy life, then you must place importance on following a healthy diet. Having a busy life is not a reason for eating unhealthy — it is an excuse. Excuses lead you to nowhere other than disappointment and regrets. Is that what you really want for yourself?

Remember, you can achieve most things in life, but only if your reason is strong enough. Finding the time to cook and eat healthy and nutritious foods is one of the reasons that many people do not find important, unfortunately.

Creating Healthy Daily Routines

A routine is a set of habits that you follow regularly. Each of your routines are made of a set of actions that you keep performing daily. The healthier the habits you create, the healthier routines you will develop. Healthy habits and healthy routines together can support you to achieve your goals and change your life, and they work together, hand in hand.

We all have a number of daily routines. They help us build a structure to our lives and create discipline. They also help us to focus on the things that are important, such as health and relationships. Daily routines add the benefits of being more organised and productive. Developing healthy routines around your meals, your exercise, and your self-care is important for your personal and professional life, whilst also helping you to feel more in control of your own day and your own life in general.

Ultimately, days filled with healthy routines promise a healthy lifestyle, which lead to a healthy life.

Creating the Environment That Works for You

To increase the chances of creating a healthy lifestyle, you need to make your environment work for you. Surround yourself with things and people that will help you move forward, and get rid of the triggers that pull you back towards the direction you do not want to go.

If you made a decision to stop indulging in chocolate, you need to make sure that your environment is chocolate-free on the days you decide not to eat it.

If you decided that your new lifestyle has to include a healthy diet, then you need to make sure that you get rid of all the junk and processed foods, and have plenty of vegetables in the fridge, a bag of nuts in your car, and some fruits in the office, etc.

If exercising is something that you want to focus on, then make your environment work for you. Having an exercise bike in your lounge or your bedroom is something that will remind you of your goal.

You can now see how your environment can affect your behaviour. It can encourage you to behave a certain way, or it can discourage you. By ensuring that you are creating an environment that is focused on encouragement and positivity, you are setting yourself up for success, rather than failure.

Whatever area of your life you want to improve and focus on, whether it is eating healthy, doing exercise, going to bed earlier, or feeling less stressed, make sure that your behaviour leads to establishing habits that are goal-oriented. Having something solid to work towards makes the whole process far easier as a result.

How to Develop the Right Mindset

At the beginning of each year, many people from all over the world try to eat healthy and regularly visit the gym in order to get healthier or lose weight. This is common behaviour for this time of the year, and as a result, gyms are doing great business!

The problem is that this sort of behaviour is not supported by any kind of understanding around nutrition or an established plan for exercising. Instead, their behaviour is dictated by a New Year's resolution. This means that their focus is not strong enough, and that by the middle of January or into February, their will to keep going to the gym will waver, and they will eventually give up, usually having to pay a full year's gym membership because they have signed themselves into a contract they now have no intention of using.

If you do not understand the real reason for your behaviour, then your willpower, motivation, and desire for success will not survive in a busy world filled with responsibilities and commitments. Without a strong reason and the right mindset, you will struggle in trying to live a healthy lifestyle when life gets too busy or too challenging.

There are four steps to success when it comes to developing the right mindset:

- Be clear about why it is important to you to lead a healthy lifestyle, and ask yourself how willing you are to eat healthy at times when people around you eat unhealthy. How willing are you to exercise when you do not feel like it, and how willing are you to stop drinking after having only one small glass of wine? Be honest with your answers, as these will give you information on areas you might need to focus on a little more than you originally thought.

- Write your answers down. Do not be shy. It is only you who will see them. No one else will have access to them, unless you want to share them with people in your life. There is no need to hide, and it is important and therapeutic for you to write down your thoughts. Writing them down will make things clearer and will highlight the meaning of your goals and desires, effectively setting them in stone.

- Make an action plan that will help you achieve your goals. Later on in the book I will give you some practical tips and ideas on how to find the time to exercise, eat healthy, stress less, and relax more. These tips will help you to create the action steps you may want to apply in your daily life to achieve your health goals.

- Keep going back to Step One, and keep reminding yourself why it is important for you to achieve this goal. This will not only help you get started, but it will help you carry on with your behaviour, which will then become a habit that will stay with you for as long as you want to keep it. Knowing your reasons will help you to stay on track when willpower leaves you and motivation deserts you. Understanding why you want to achieve your goal will help your mindset to join your behaviour, and together they will help you create the life you want.

It is important to remember that your health and weight do not depend only on your diet. This is something many people believe, but it actually comes down to a variety of different factors, including your activity levels, stress levels, your happiness, and your biology. These elements play an important role in determining how well the diet you follow will work, the way your body processes the food you eat, and whether your diet can keep your body in good order.

This also depends on your age, gender, hormones, stress, digestive system, muscle mass, the speed of your metabolism, etc. They all work together and constantly interact with each other.

You are unable to influence some of these factors, such as your age and gender, but you are always in control of what you eat, how physically active you are, and what kind of lifestyle you lead. The choices you make on an everyday basis can have a positive or negative impact on your life, your health, and your body.

I understand that people with physical restrictions, especially those who are unable to walk, are limited to do certain activities; therefore, they are less in control and not always able to choose activities they would like to do. But please remember that we are all in control of how we respond to the circumstances we live in. Focusing on the positive will bring positive change, and focusing on the negative will bring negative change. The right mindset can help us to overcome the most difficult hurdles we face.

In the next section, we are going to look at how you can develop a healthy morning routine to help you start the day the right way. By developing a healthy morning routine, you will be one step closer to living a healthy life.

How to Develop a Healthy Morning Routine

The way you start your day has a huge say in how the rest of it is going to continue. Your morning routine helps you to kick-start the day in a healthy manner. It sets the tone for the day and improves productivity. What you do within the first couple of hours of getting up in the morning can affect your mood and performance for the rest of the day, and take it in either a positive direction or a negative one.

Studies suggest that the quality of your morning routine determines the quality of your day. Creating a healthy structure to your morning routine can help you set the pace for the hours ahead, improve your health, life, and general well-being. It can make you feel more confident, energised, and improve your health and life in so many ways. However, if you start your day in the wrong way, the rest of the hours, until bedtime, are likely to continue in the same way, and you will find yourself lacking energy, being quite unproductive, and probably suffering from low mood or general agitation too.

As such, the way you start the day is often the way you will finish the day, and this is the reason why developing a healthy morning routine is so important. Focusing on healthy habits in the morning will often trigger more healthy habits and healthy behaviours during the day. So, when you start the day with the intention to be positive, you will find that the rest of the day is more likely to be positive too. It is a silent intention that works very well indeed.

5 Healthy Morning Habits

In this section, I would like to talk about my favourite morning habits that I do regularly, and I suggest that you implement them in your morning routine too. If some do not make sense to you, tweak them into something that you can implement to make it a little easier for your own needs. There are many habits that I could include in the list, but these five habits are a good starting point to help you begin the day in a healthy way, and they are the ones that I use on a regular basis.

Stay Hydrated

Drinking water helps your body to stay hydrated after not consuming any foods and drinks for several hours during the night. Having a glass of water with a slice of lemon soon after you get up in the morning, will help your digestive system to function smoothly, and fuel your brain.

Make Time for a Healthy Breakfast

It is not only important to have a breakfast, but to have a healthy breakfast, and fill your body with the right nutrients at the start of the day. Having a healthy breakfast will provide you with a boost of energy, and will positively affect your health and well-being.

Including protein in your breakfast will increase satiety and give you energy until lunchtime. In the third chapter of this book, I will share with you what a healthy breakfast consists of, to give you some ideas of how you can fuel yourself up with the first meal of the day.

Move Your Body

Doing exercise first thing in the morning is good for you for many reasons. Morning exercise can sharpen your brain and make you feel more alert. After exercising, you will feel more energised and be ready for the day ahead. Morning exercise can speed up your metabolism, so if your aim is to lose weight, then doing morning exercise is a great habit to have.

One of the benefits of a fast metabolism is that it helps to burn calories faster, and this can help your weight loss progress. Studies suggest that exercising before breakfast, on an empty stomach after fasting during the night, can help you burn more fat.

Exercise also helps with stress, because it releases a hormone called dopamine in your brain. This is a hormone that boosts your mood and helps you to start your day feeling happy and positive.

In Chapter Four, we are going to talk more about exercising, and explore how you can find the time and motivation to exercise, or simply to move more during the day.

Be Grateful

I suggest you start the day with positive thoughts, and gratitude is one of them. It is such a healthy emotion, so be sure to include it in your everyday life. Be grateful for the things you have, and make your first thought of the day a positive one. Expressing gratitude helps rewire your brain, and makes you feel more positive about your life in general. You are the only one who is in control of your thoughts, so make them work for you, rather than against you.

Listen to Uplifting Music or Watch a Motivational Video on YouTube

This is my favourite habit, which I have developed over the last couple of years. Listening to uplifting music or watching a motivational video will lift your spirits, helping you to feel inspired and more alive as you start the day. This will reduce stress and increase happiness.

You can do this while you are brushing your teeth, getting dressed, doing your morning exercise, or having breakfast. It is very easy to implement it into your morning routine. It does not require much effort from your part, and it helps you feel more positive about the day ahead.

As already discussed, for healthy habits to become a part of your morning routine, they need to be repeated numerous times. Remember, you are aiming for your healthy habits to be done on autopilot. The more you repeat them, the easier it will be to do them, and the more you will enjoy doing them.

Here are the steps to follow that can help you develop the healthy morning habits I have mentioned in this section, or you can choose your own if you prefer:

- When you wake up each morning, make a conscious decision to start working on your new habit.
- Choose one of the healthy morning habits I mentioned, choosing the one you feel most comfortable to start working on first.
- Carry on working on your new habit until you do it on autopilot. It might take you a few weeks of repetitive behaviour before it starts feeling easier, or even a few months before your new behaviour becomes a habit. It does not matter how long it takes you, but working on developing your new habit will help you get closer to where you want to be.
- When your chosen action becomes a habit, move on to another action, and work towards another habit that can become a part of your routine.

By focusing on following healthy actions every morning, you will notice a difference in the way you feel, think, and the way you behave for the rest of the day.

Developing a healthy morning routine is equally as important as developing a healthy bedtime routine. They can both help you to feel healthier and more positive. This is something I am going to talk about in the next section, where we explore how you can develop a bedtime routine and what benefits you can experience by doing so.

How to Develop a Healthy Bedtime Routine

Getting enough sleep is essential for good health; it enables the body to repair, reduces stress, helps concentration, and reduces the risk of heart disease and stroke. The correct amount varies a little from person to person, but generally it is between six and eight hours a night.

Sadly, many people nowadays get neither the amount nor the quality of sleep they need. Sometimes this is due to medical conditions such as apnoea, but more often it is a lifestyle issue. So, what can you do to improve your sleep?

Making sure you have a good night's sleep is an important part of a healthy lifestyle, and having a healthy bedtime routine can help you improve your quality of sleep. It has been proven that sleep improves memory, reduces stress, and refuels the mind and body. A healthy bedtime routine can prepare your body and mind for a good night's sleep.

To help you out, here are some tips and suggestions on how you can improve your bedtime routine.

Timing Is Crucial

The first thing to look at is timing. This is crucial, as the best way of ensuring a good night's sleep is to keep to the same timing every night, as much as possible. Start by determining when you need to wake up in the morning, calculate back from there when you need to go to sleep, and set that as your bedtime.

It is important that you stick to this timetable. It can be tempting to stay in bed late at the weekend, or if you have slept badly, but this is only going to throw your body clock off and make it harder to establish a regular sleep pattern.

Plan Your Day the Night Before

You will not waste any time in the morning if you already made plans the night before. This includes taking clothes out of the wardrobe, ready to be worn in the morning. It also includes leaving a pair of trainers by the front door, so that you are ready for your morning workout. Basically, make it easier for yourself to start your day in the right way, by doing what you can the night before when you are naturally higher in energy.

Making a list of what needs to be done the following day, physically or mentally (writing it on a piece of paper is usually more helpful), can make you more productive the next day. The act of writing it down also solidifies it in your mind, so you are less likely to forget something important.

I suggest you spend under five minutes on making plans for the next day, and I do not want you to stress over it. You already know what needs to be done, what appointments you need to attend, or phone calls you need to make. However, planning and scheduling will give structure to your day and help you to find extra time you did not know you had.

Do Not Make It Hard for Yourself

Eating the wrong types of food late at night can keep you awake, so make sure you give yourself several hours between dinner and sleep. If you need a late-night snack, make sure it is something that is not going to give you indigestion.

Having a large, simple-carbohydrate meal before bedtime is likely to increase your blood sugar levels, followed by a sudden drop of your blood sugar levels. This imbalance will possibly affect your sleep and wake you up the middle of the night, due to the increased level of cortisol.

If you are hungry before going to bed, make sure you eat a small meal and consume the type of foods that will not affect your sleep, such as a handful of berries, or a small slice of wholemeal bread with peanut butter.

In addition, you should be mindful of what you drink, and stay away from stimulants, including coffee or fizzy drinks such as Coke or Fanta. Any caffeinated drink is likely to disrupt your sleep, but I also suggest you avoid alcohol late at night. Alcohol can help you get to sleep initially, but you will not sleep well. When the effects of alcohol wear off, it is likely you will wake in the middle of the night, or have a hangover the next morning. You may feel dehydrated or unwell, which is not a great way to start the day, and it is likely to make the rest of the day carry on in the same way.

It is important to have a winding-down process before you go to bed. Taking a warm bath will help you relax, while reading or playing easy listening music or the radio will prepare you for sleep. However, it is best to avoid smartphones or other electronic devices for a couple of hours before going to bed. These will only cause you to be more alert before bed, which is not conducive to deep relaxation and sleep. It can be very easy to lay in bed with your phone, scrolling through social media, but this is something you should try your best to avoid.

Put simply, and as much as possible, try to avoid having anything in your bedroom that is not to do with sleeping, and that certainly includes a TV. Invest in heavy curtains and soundproofing, or else use a white-noise device, to avoid being disturbed by light or noise. The more you arrange your bedroom with the sole aim of getting a good night's sleep, the more likely you are to get what you are aiming towards.

Some people also find weighted blankets to be useful for helping them both fall asleep and maintain sleep, while they may struggle with this otherwise. Weighted blankets are often used for people with restless legs syndrome (RLS), but they can simply be a sleeping aid too.

The weight of the blanket varies, so this is something you will need to experiment with until you find the product for you. Ultimately, the weight is thought to help your brain release the oxytocin hormone, as well as dopamine. This is because the weight actually feels a little like a hug. This is a relaxing hormone too, so it can therefore help you to fall asleep.

Exercise is good, of course, but exercising too close to bedtime might keep you awake. For this reason, I suggest you take exercise earlier in the day. Meditation before bedtime can also help you relax. Meditating only for a few minutes before sleep can calm you down and help you to sleep better and deeper. Many people also like soaking in an Epsom salt bath before retiring to bed. This helps them relax muscles and loosen stiff joints.

It is really about experimenting and finding a routine that suits you best and which helps you to fall asleep quickly and stay asleep until the morning. If you regularly struggle with insomnia, and you find that it is not being helped by any self-help methods, such as the ones I have mentioned above, perhaps a chat with your doctor might help you to find a solution to your problem.

Making sure that you have good quality sleep, needs to be one of your main priorities. A good night's sleep looks after your body and protects your mental health. Waking up refreshed in the morning will make you feel more energised and much happier. You will be more productive, and this will create more time in your day, whilst also ensuring that you have the willpower to avoid falling back into unhealthy habits.

Key Points

- A habit is a behaviour that has been repeated numbers of times for a longer period of time and is done on autopilot. This behaviour plays an important role in your daily life.
- Healthy habits are the source of a healthy body and a healthy mind.

- Habits are not fixed. You can change them any time you want. You are in full control of them.
- When actions are repeated numbers of times, they become habits. A set of habits create routine. Routines you follow determine the quality of your lifestyle. The healthier the routine, the healthier the lifestyle.
- The way you start the day is important. Your morning routine affects your performance during the day.
- When you wake up each morning, make a conscious decision to start working on your new habit.
- Getting enough sleep and having a healthy bedtime routine is crucial for your health and well-being.
- Plan the day the night before, and remember to wind down before bedtime. Choose to do activities that relax you. Healthy bedtime routines can help you slow down and prepare you for a good night's sleep.

Chapter 2: Diet

"A healthy diet is a solution to many of our health-care problems. It is the most important solution."

John Mackey

How to Find the Diet That Works

There are lots of different diets and a variety of opinions on what the best diet is. So many options tend to bring confusion, and I am aware that lots of people go from one diet to another, searching for that miracle diet that works; the one that helps with weight loss, the one that can slow down the ageing process, the one that can support arthritis, or heart issues, or diabetes. The truth is that there is no magic fix.

What we choose to eat can affect our health and our whole life. As Ann Wigmore said," *The food you eat can be either the safest and most powerful form of medicine or the slowest form of poison."*

But why do we have so many diets?

All diets have their unique rules and guidance. They all try to teach us what is healthy and what we should be eating. But not all diets are considered to be healthy. Diets that promise a quick weight loss are known as "fad diets" and should be avoided. These are often unsustainable, leave you feeling miserable, and cut out important food groups which can damage health and well-being, rather than being at all useful. In addition, the weight you lose on these diets is extremely likely to return the moment you stop following the diet.

Some diets tend to be influenced by personal or cultural beliefs. Examples of these include vegetarian, ketogenic, and vegan diets. Other diets are ruled by spiritual or religious beliefs, such as a halal or kosher diet.

In Western culture and the busy world we live in, most diets are impacted by bad habits or the desire to lose weight. With the huge choice of diets on the market, it is not surprising that most people find it confusing to understand which diet to follow.

Over the years people have followed a number of diets in order to lose weight, such as a low fat diet, low calorie diet, grapefruit diet, cabbage soup diet, South Beach diet, Weight Watchers diet, etc. Popular diets that offer some health benefits are intermittent fasting, ketogenic diet, Mediterranean diet, Paleo diet, GI diet, and low GL diet. There are also many other diets, but these diets are not crash diets. They embrace the way of eating that can provide health benefits, if followed properly. None of these diets are focused on counting calories but on prioritising certain foods over others.

In the case of intermittent fasting, the focus is on cycling between eating and fasting over a certain period of time. I am not favouring one diet over another. I am also not recommending you follow any particular diet right now, as the purpose of this book is to show you how you can eat healthy and live a healthy life despite being busy, so that you can feel empowered to make healthy dietary and lifestyle choices that can benefit you the most.

So, what works?

Most people have an idea of what a healthy diet consists of, but not many people follow their own advice. As I already mentioned, there are many diets on the market, and I have noticed that people are often trying to follow famous diets, even though most of them do not produce long-term results, instead of simply eating healthy.

I understand that the idea of a healthy diet is different for each person, but the basic principles are always the same — eat plenty of fruits, veggies, and foods containing fibre, and avoid simple carbohydrates and eating late at night. Do not deprive yourself of the foods you love, and allow yourself to have occasional treats. Moderation is the key. This is as simple as it needs to be.

My advice is that whenever you follow any kind of diet, have your health in mind. Diets that are designed only to assist you in losing weight are unhealthy and often unsustainable. I strongly advise against them, but those that promote health can help you reach and maintain a healthy weight, as well as support your overall well-being. It is about finding a route that works for you and one that you can sustain over the long term. Remember, becoming healthier is about making healthy, life-long changes.

How to Eat the Right Way

Proteins, carbohydrates, and fats are the three macronutrients essential in the human diet. Each of them plays a vital role in keeping the body healthy. Vitamins and minerals, known as micronutrients, are equally important for good functioning of the body, but they are needed in much smaller amounts. I am briefly going to discuss each macronutrient so you have some understanding of their roles and the importance of including them in your diet. This will also help you understand why fad diets simply do not work and are not at all healthy.

Carbohydrates

The first macronutrient that I want to talk about is carbohydrates. Many people try to reduce eating them, and the main reason for this is often because of the belief that carbohydrates will make them put weight on. However, did you know that carbohydrates can be found in most foods?

You can even find them in fruits and vegetables. It is about good and bad in many ways, not simply cutting out any carb.

I want you to understand that not all carbohydrates are the same, and the body digests them differently; therefore, they affect the body in different ways.

Your body needs complex carbohydrates as they provide your body with energy. They can be found in whole grains, legumes, and most fruits and vegetables. Complex carbohydrates are rich in fibre, and the body digests them more slowly. Therefore, they provide you with energy for a longer period of time.

You should reduce consumption of simple carbohydrates. They are found in white bread, white pasta, and white rice. These foods have been heavily processed and tend to raise your blood sugar levels. This gives you an instant spike of energy followed by the sudden crush, making you feel lethargic.

Sugar is a type of carbohydrate that I recommend you avoid. Sugar contributes to weight gain and causes many diseases. You can find sugar in breakfast cereals, soft drinks, low fat yoghurts, cakes, biscuits, many sauces, etc.

Fats

So many people are absolutely petrified of eating fats. The traditional view is that fat is bad for us and should be avoided in a healthy diet. However, while some types of fat can increase the risk of obesity and heart disease, other types are essential for healthy eating, and can even help us to lose weight. Eating healthy fats gives us energy, regulates body temperature, protects the organs, and helps us absorb vitamins.

There are different types of fats: trans fat, saturated fat, and unsaturated fat. Trans fat is the one that needs to be avoided. It can be found in very small quantities in meat and dairy, but it is mainly synthetic and is found in fried and processed foods, as well as in cakes and biscuits.

Saturated fat is present in meat, eggs, fish, and dairy, as well as in coconut oil and almond oil. In the past, we were told that saturated fat is bad for our health, but findings from recent years suggest otherwise and claim that saturated fats are good for us. Unsaturated fats can be found in olive oil, nuts, and tofu. They are also present in oily fish, such as salmon, trout, and tuna. These foods should make up a significant part of a healthy diet.

Proteins

Along with carbohydrates and fats, proteins are essential for our diet. They play a number of important roles in keeping us healthy. Proteins build new muscle and other tissues. They also repair the wear and tear that the body suffers, as well as playing a significant role in a weight-loss diet.

The biggest enemy on a weight-loss journey is hunger. This gives rise to cravings, but a protein-rich diet can help reduce this effect. This is because proteins affect the hormones that control your hunger. If you replace carbohydrate and fat with protein, you will reduce the hunger hormone and boost satiety hormones.

Eating protein also keeps your blood sugar stable, which regulates your hunger levels. In addition to all of this, the muscles the proteins build will help keep you fitter, stronger, and feeling more positive about yourself.

Proteins are usually associated with meat, fish, and dairy, but there are also many excellent plant-based sources of protein, including nuts, pulses, soya, and some green vegetables.

In order to keep your blood sugar levels stable, which is the key to good health, I suggest you add protein to every meal you eat. This will help you manage your hunger, and reduce your cravings for sugary snacks.

Vitamins and Minerals

Vitamins and minerals are needed in smaller quantities, but they are equally important for the health of the body, the same as macronutrients. They play many vital roles in the body, such as keeping our skin and hair healthy or protecting our immune system.

There are 13 essential vitamins and over 100 minerals. They all offer different benefits to our body and play different, but very significant, roles. You can find vitamins and minerals in fruits and vegetables but also in meat, fish, and dairy products.

How to Eat a Variety of Foods and Why

Healthy eating cannot be achieved from any one food or any few. There are good reasons to make sure you have a varied diet. There are many foods that contain nutrients vital to a healthy diet, but no single food contains everything you need.

For example, lean meat or nuts are excellent sources of protein but not vitamin C; whereas you can get vitamin C from oranges, but they are not a good protein source. Since both are vital for your health, neither works on its own.

This can be multiplied through the dozens of nutrients we require, and you need to find sources for each of them. Besides the broad needs, such as proteins to build muscle and carbs to produce energy, the many vitamins, minerals, and other chemicals in food have specific functions. Ensuring a balanced intake of them all will help you maintain a healthy body, including (vitally) a healthy gut.

There are six main food groups:

- Proteins – These come from meat, fish, and dairy, as well as from beans, nuts and soya.
- Vegetables – As we have previously seen, it is vital to get a wide variety of vegetables by *eating the rainbow*.
- Fruit – This too comes in a rainbow of colours, all important for a balanced diet.
- Grains, rice, and pasta – These should be wholegrain wherever possible.

- Dairy or equivalent – These should include milk, cheese, and yoghurt, or non-dairy alternatives such as soya or coconut milk.
- Fats and oils – You need a certain amount of these in your diet, but avoid eating trans fats as they are damaging to your health.

I would love to give you some ideas about how to ensure that you eat a variety of foods. Even when you are struggling with time, eating a variety of foods should not be difficult; most supermarkets stock a huge range. The problem can be motivation. It is always easier just to stick to what we know.

A few strategies can get you experimenting more, and broadening your diet. The simplest way is to set yourself the goal of trying something new every week. As long as it is healthy, it does not matter which of the food groups it is from, although it would be useful to target a different group each week. If you enjoy it, it can simply become part of your regular shopping list.

Looking around for new recipes to use can suggest ingredients you have never used before. TV is flooded with cooking programmes, and they all show the ingredients list and cooking method of different dishes to cook. The internet is another place to look for new recipes, learn new dishes, and experiment with cooking foods that you have never tried before. There are a number of dishes that can be cooked in 20 minutes or less. There is really no excuse for not learning to cook new dishes and using different ingredients at least once per week.

We also need to talk about another diet-related subject: the importance of eating the rainbow. I am sure you have heard numerous times that you should eat a variety of colours. Why is this important, you might ask? Because each colour offers different benefits to your body.

Perhaps one of the stranger pieces of nutritional advice, on the face of it, is the advice to eat foods with as wide a range of colours as possible. This is not just for aesthetic reasons, however. Provided the colour of a plant-based food is natural, it can actually give a strong clue about its nutritional character.

Plants contain a wide range of phytochemicals, which perform various functions in protecting them or aiding their growth. The important thing for our purposes, though, is that each of these phytochemicals is rich in a different selection of the vitamins and minerals essential to our diet.

Since it is these phytochemicals that control the colour of the fruit or vegetable derived from the plant, this makes colour a useful guide to the nutritional value of the food. It is not absolute, but "eating the rainbow" provides a simple way of ensuring you are getting a good balanced diet.
So, what do the different colours show?

- Red fruits and vegetables are rich in vitamins A and C, as well as phytochemicals such as lycopene, and have been associated with a decrease in the risk of some cancers. Examples are tomatoes, red peppers, strawberries, cherries, and beets.

- Orange and yellow fruits and vegetables are also good sources of vitamins A and C, as well as the phytonutrient hesperidin, and are associated with an improved immune system and a lower risk of heart disease. Examples are oranges, carrots, peaches, sweet potatoes, and orange/yellow peppers.
- Green fruits and vegetables are a good source of vitamin K, which promotes blood and bone health, as well as a number of other nutrients. They have been associated with an improved immune system and mood enhancement. Examples are broccoli, kiwi fruit, kale, spinach, and peas.
- Blue and purple fruits and vegetables are rich in vitamins C and K, as well as a number of phytonutrients, and appear to have anti-inflammatory properties. Examples are blueberries, aubergine, red cabbage (which is actually purple), and plums.
- White and brown fruits, vegetables, and fungi contain vitamins C, K, and B9, and a range of important phytonutrients that are good for the bones and the heart, as well as having been associated with a reduced risk of some cancers. Examples are mushrooms, garlic, potatoes, cauliflower, and onions.

Ensuring that you include a variety of colours in your diet is vital for your overall health. The vitamins, minerals, and phytochemicals indicated by the various colours of foods play crucial roles in your body's healthy functioning.

While you could analyse the contents of each food, it is far easier just to eat the rainbow. And it is far more fun. Whichever way you approach it, be adventurous. In the end, your health will benefit and you might even discover foods that you really like, that you never knew existed before.

How to Eat Healthy When You Do Not Have Time

The way healthy eating advice is often given, you would be forgiven for thinking that it is a full-time job, and that you must have plenty of time to do everything exactly right. Of course, you do not. The reality is that you often will not have time to plan and prepare healthy meals as you would like, and the temptation then is to give up and phone for a takeaway.

There are alternatives, though. Even if your meals are not perfect on those days, they can still be healthy. Approaching your meals with a healthy mindset does not always have to follow every one of the rules, as long as the willingness is there, and you are doing your best to at least improve the nutritional content of what you are eating for that particular meal.

Planning ahead helps prevent unhealthy spontaneity, and whilst it seems counter-intuitive, careful planning allows you to be both better prepared and more flexible and adaptable for your meals. You are better prepared because, if you have drawn up your menus and done your weekly shop based on them, you can go straight into making the meal you planned. This saves you time and stops you having to think about what you are going to eat for dinner that day.

On the other hand, you can be even better prepared by building up a stock of alternative recipes, including some quick and easy ones, and knowing which ones you can make with similar ingredients. That way, if you arrive home too exhausted or too rushed to make what you had intended, you will know what you can do quickly and easily instead.

Sometimes, especially when you are busy and rushing through the day, it is important to compromise on the ingredients. Yes, in an ideal world we would like to cook only with fresh ingredients bought that day; in practice, this is neither always possible nor essential. Many short-cuts are still reasonably healthy, including:

- Frozen vegetables
- Pre-chopped vegetables
- Pre-marinated meat
- Prepared sauces
- Tinned food

Of course, this requires doing due diligence when you are shopping. Check the labels for all ingredients, especially any additives, and go for low-salt varieties, as well as ensuring that prepared or frozen meat and vegetables come from the best sources. Having your cupboards and freezer stocked up with these options will help you pick a quick alternative meal.

Here are my recommendations for how you can eat healthy even if you are a busy mum, a busy full-time working person, or a parent taking care of a large family.

Cook in Bulk

This will save you plenty of time. If you are pressed for time, cook only once a week. Choose one evening per week to cook two or three different dishes. Cook large amounts of foods and freeze them for the evenings when you do not have much time to do any cooking. Cooking in bulk will give you the opportunity to have a home cooked meal every night of the week.

Leftovers Are Good

Again, it is good to prepare a new meal from scratch each time, but it is not essential. Whether leftovers are accidental or deliberate, they can be repurposed. Of course, there are items that do not last well after being cooked, but for the most part, extra meat or vegetables can be incorporated into a future recipe.

On the other hand, you can pre-empt not having time by getting into the habit of sometimes cooking more than you need, and freezing what is left over. That means you will have something quick, easy, and healthy to reach for when you need it.

Are these options ideal? Not necessarily, but we are not living in an ideal world. Also, they will enable you to eat a reasonably healthy meal instead of turning to takeaways.

Shopping List

Doing internet shopping and having food delivered to your door is ideal for busy people. When doing shopping, whether you do your food shopping on the internet or you physically go to the shop to buy your food, have a shopping list ready. You will not waste time searching for the items you want to buy, and you will not become tempted to buy anything that you do not need.

Having a list ready will help you to be more disciplined, and you will stick to buying only the foods that are on your list. If you think that you do not have time to do a shopping list, then think again; how about doing it while travelling on the train to work, or while relaxing in front of the TV in the evening. Remember, a shopping list can be done only once per week, and once you get into the habit of doing it, you will need less than 10 minutes to do it.

Eating healthy when you do not have time is sometimes just a mind game. If you convince yourself that you are too busy for eating healthy, then you will never find time to cook and eat healthy meals. I understand that it is sometimes much easier and quicker to put some chips in the oven or have a microwave meal, but taking a prepared home-cooked meal out of the freezer in the morning, and eating it in the evening, is probably less time and energy consuming. If you always come up with excuses why you cannot, or should not, do something, then maybe what you want is not what you really want.

If you are always finding excuses for not having time to eat healthy, or to do anything that will improve your health, then you need to ask yourself how much you really want it. Developing a new relationship with food is important if you want to start eating healthy. This goes hand in hand with developing a new attitude towards self-care, which will help you to improve your health, your well-being, and your quality of life. We are going to explore this further, later on in the book; but for now, let's stay focused on your diet and how you can improve it.

How to Eat Your Favourite Foods Without Depriving Yourself

One of the foremost reasons why people fail in their attempts to eat healthy or to lose weight, and keep it off, is that they make it hard for themselves. They adopt an "all or nothing" mentality, and they concentrate on dieting instead of eating healthy. When this happens, their way of eating becomes a chore that they cannot keep up. This is not only bad for their weight loss goals, but also for their mental health. This is an unhealthy way of thinking, which often brings negative results and leads to perceived failure.

The problem with most diets is that they are based on you having to tell yourself "I must not eat this or that food." The result, especially if it is something you particularly enjoy, is that you cannot stop thinking about it, and sooner or later, you are going to give in and have that chocolate cake or those chips. When this happens, you tend to eat a large quantity of the foods that you deprived yourself of.

Have you ever noticed this? So, instead of having one chocolate bar, you have two or three. And instead of having one pizza, you may have two, or have garlic bread for a starter and a large piece of cheesecake for dessert in addition to having pizza as the main meal. In the moment, it feels amazing, but quickly afterwards, the guilt sets in, and in some cases it can be crushing.

Of course, in reality, this is not a big deal, as long as it does not happen often; but if your diet is based on "I must not," you are likely to feel a failure, and this can be damaging. This may lower your self-esteem, which not only damages your general mental health but also makes it harder to stick to your diet.

Eating healthy instead of dieting is the key. Instead of a diet that tells you what you must not eat, it is far better to concentrate on identifying the foods that are good for you. Do not think of it as "I must not eat sugary cereal," but as "I choose to eat oats with nuts and fresh fruit." Giving yourself permission to have a treat every now and again, makes it far more likely that you will stick to your eating plan and then treat yourself occasionally, rather than treating yourself constantly, and failing in your healthy eating attempts.

In most cases, if you have chosen the healthy food, you are likely to find that you enjoy it at least as much as your old choices. Do not force yourself too hard, though, as there is usually an alternative. For instance, spinach is good for you, but if you really cannot stand spinach, then do not eat it. Find another vegetable with a similar nutritional value, that you do enjoy. There is a huge range out there, so you are sure to find something.

Start implementing your dietary changes slowly. One of the ways to do this is to add something healthy to your unhealthy food. A good example is pizza. Instead of having your usual pepperoni pizza, the healthy alternative could be a vegetable pizza. Adding fresh healthy ingredients to your pizza is a good starting point towards healthy eating. You are making slow progress, with baby steps, and these baby steps are always better than not taking any steps at all.

In addition, did you know that treats are actually good for you? As I mentioned earlier, having the occasional unhealthy food item is not going to do you too much harm, as long as it is occasional. The best way to ensure this is to make it deliberate — give yourself permission to have treats, instead of seeing it as going astray.

One approach is to give yourself a 10% window each day to treat yourself to an unhealthy favourite food. You do not have to use it, of course, and the chances are that the more you enjoy eating healthy foods, the less you will actually want to eat unhealthy treats.

I often notice this happening with people whose aim is to lose weight. After successfully losing some weight, they do not want to go back to their old habits and indulge in the food they used to love. After developing a habit of eating healthy, most people ultimately start to enjoy it.

If you start by enjoying the prospect of feeling healthy and looking great, rather than setting yourself prohibitions, you will soon start to find that you are enjoying the healthy food too. When you enjoy the way you feel, you will make sure you find the time and energy to look after your body.

How to Make Sure You Drink More Water

The single most important item in your diet is water. That is hardly surprising, since your body is made up of about 60% water, which is around 2/3 of your body weight, and this needs to be constantly replenished.

Water is vital for everything from brain activity to skin tone, so it is disturbing that statistics suggest that most people do not drink nearly enough water. In fact, some appear to drink none at all, putting their health at serious risk.

Why do we need water?

Almost every process in your body requires water to function correctly, which means that dehydration can have serious consequences. The blood that carries oxygen and nutrients around your body is 90% water, and without enough water, it becomes thicker, raising your blood pressure.

Water also supports the functioning of your brain and neural system, so brain function will decline without enough water. Dehydration can also lead to kidney disease, digestive problems, and joint pains, among other things.

However, on the flip side, drinking enough water can increase performance during exercise, improve the health of your skin, and even aid in weight loss. Drinking plenty of water can also help with constipation.

Some people claim that drinking water before they eat makes them feel full and less likely to overeat. Several studies suggest that middle-aged and older adults experience weight loss when drinking water before each meal, and one study showed that those drinking water before the meal saw 44% more weight loss compared to a group of people who did not drink water before their meals.

But how much water do you need daily?

There are different opinions on this and, over the years, many studies have been done on this topic. The general advice is to drink 8 glasses or 2 litres of water each day. A report published in the early years of the 21st century claims that men should be drinking 3.7 litres daily, and women should drink 2.7 litres per day. These are approximate figures, and it is suggested that the right amount of water depends on our age and weight, as well as the requirements of the individual. During hot weather, it is likely that water intake will have to increase, as well as during exercising, or if we suffer from a fever, vomit, or have diarrhoea.

Hydration can come from various sources. Some foods can be a good source of water, including various fruits, vegetables, and salads. Here is a list of the individual foods that are very high in water content, and I suggest you include these foods in your diet:

- Cucumbers
- Tomatoes
- Spinach
- Mushrooms
- Melon
- Broccoli
- Brussel sprouts
- Oranges
- Apples
- Blueberries
- Strawberries

These foods not only have high water content and help you stay hydrated, but they also provide you with fibre and various vitamins and minerals, all playing an important role in keeping your body healthy and contributing to your daily water intake.

Despite the fact that you get water from food, sometimes it is simply not enough to fulfil the needs of your body. As a result, I encourage you to make sure that you drink plenty of water and always stay hydrated as a first rule.

Drinking water needs to become a habit, so if you have trouble remembering, it is important to consciously form that habit. Start by keeping a log of each time you drink water during the day, and estimate how much you have drunk. When you are regularly hitting your target, you have formed the habit.

It is also a good idea to make sure there is always water available. Having a water filter jug at home will help you keep track of how much water you are drinking, as well as providing high quality water. Always carry a water bottle with you when you are out, and not just when it is hot or when you are exercising. Having a water bottle on you will remind you to regularly sip water during the day.

Above all, learn to appreciate water; it is the healthiest drink of them all.

How to Develop a Healthy Approach to Weight Loss

If you have decided to take losing weight seriously, your first reaction might be to go on a crash diet, obsessively counting calories and reducing your intake to the lowest level possible. You probably will lose weight, but there are two big problems: You could damage your health, and you are likely to put the weight straight back on.

While portion control is important, the vital thing for healthy weight loss is to plan and eat a well-balanced diet. This means including healthy options from all the main food groups. For example:

- Protein from fish, lean meat, or legumes
- Carbohydrates from wholemeal grains, rice, or starchy vegetables

- A wide range of vegetables, salads, and fruit
- Milk and dairy, or an equivalent

Each of these food groups is vital for your well-being, and a diet that urges you to cut out any of them is unlikely to be good for your health. On the other hand, food or drink with high sugar content offers little nutritional value and will damage your attempt to lose weight. These items should be kept for occasional treats.

As much as possible (I understand that it is not always possible), prepare meals with fresh ingredients, and avoid ready meals and fast food. Apart from being healthier, it means you know exactly what has gone into your meals. If you are going to eat out, choose a venue you trust to prepare healthy food.

Here are a few tips for a healthy diet as part of a healthy lifestyle:

- Do not skip meals in order to keep your calorie intake down. It is both healthier and more effective to eat smaller portions regularly.
- Drink plenty of water – It is healthy and will fill you up, so you will want to eat less.
- Limit your alcohol intake – Plan what you are going to allow yourself as a reward.
- Get plenty of sleep, and keep your sleep pattern regular.
- Exercise regularly, whether it is in the gym or just sometimes leaving the car at home.

- Do not be too hard on yourself. Allowing yourself occasional treats might actually help you stay on course.

One of the biggest problems with dieting, particularly fad diets, is that once the diet is over, the fat gradually creeps back. Eventually, you are back to square one and feeling thoroughly depressed. Yes, you could go back on the diet, but you no longer have confidence in your ability to achieve your goal.

It is a short-term strategy that can ultimately be self-destructive. If you want to lose weight for good, you need a different mindset.

What you tell yourself will make a substantial difference to the outcome. If you tell yourself that you are "on a diet," that implies something that has an end. You may even find yourself looking forward to finishing the diet, and that can be a dangerous state of mind for when you are no longer imposing restrictions on yourself.

Instead of dieting, it is more productive to think in terms of changing your life. You are not forbidding yourself certain foods as some kind of penance. You are taking the decision that from now on you are going to eat healthier, because it is going to make you feel great.

Setting more positive, longer-term goals will be a natural consequence of this change. The primary aim is no longer to lose X amount of weight (although that is still important) but to be more healthy.

The trigger that makes you decide to lose weight may be to fit into a favourite dress or pair of jeans again, or to look great on the beach, but that should not be the ultimate goal. Once you have achieved it, you have left yourself with no incentive to carry on keeping the weight off. Instead, it is better to focus on what it will feel like to be healthy. It is easier to stick with internal goals, such as being healthy or having more energy, than external ones, such as how others will see you.

Many diets are short-term not only because they have a natural limit, but also because they make demands that would be difficult to maintain for long. That is largely because they are based on forbidding desirable foods and making you feel guilty for any failings.

A successful approach to weight loss is obtained through healthy eating, and focuses on the benefits the healthy foods will give you. The main focus is not on losing X amount of weight by starving yourself or following fad diets. Also, because it is a long-term strategy, you can afford to be flexible. If you could not resist that cake this week, never mind; you are still mostly eating healthy, and the occasional detour is not the end of the world.

In the end, healthy eating is its own reward. As the health benefits kick in alongside the weight loss, you will start to wonder what you ever saw in junk food and sugary drinks. And that is the best guarantee that your weight loss will be for good.

Losing weight can be hard work, which makes it discouraging that only 20% of people who achieve their weight-loss target succeed in keeping the weight off long-term. The reality is that losing weight is only half the battle — maintaining a healthy weight is the real challenge.

There tends to be three main reasons why people fail to maintain their weight loss:

- The nature of the diet — very low-calorie intake can slow the metabolism and encourage the body to store more fat
- Thinking of the diet as a quick fix, rather than a long-term change in lifestyle
- Following rules based on willpower, rather than building sustainable habits into your lifestyle

When planning your weight-loss journey, it is important to develop a healthy lifestyle that you can live with. The majority of people fail during the maintenance phase because their new lifestyle is not something they can sustain for a long time. For this reason, maintaining a healthy weight after a successful weight loss is often a struggle for so many people.

A weight-maintenance diet may not be identical to a weight-loss diet, but it follows the same principles. Eat regular meals consisting of a balance of the essential nutrients, ensuring that they come from healthy sources, e.g. wholegrains rather than processed carbs, and healthy fats rather than trans fat.

Make sure you eat plenty of healthy protein too, since this boosts the hormones that tell us we have eaten enough, reducing the risk of overeating. Avoid skipping meals (especially breakfast), and drink plenty of water. Similarly, working 30 minutes of exercise into your daily routine is far more likely to help you maintain your weight than occasionally dedicating an entire day to it. Besides the exercise burning off excess calories, it will also increase your metabolism, giving the food you eat less chance to be stored as fat.

Maintaining a healthy weight is not just something you do while you are eating or exercising. Your lifestyle can make a significant difference. Having a healthy lifestyle is important in maintaining your healthy weight.

Getting enough sleep, for instance, is as vital for weight maintenance as for your general health. This is partly because sleep deprivation creates a hormone imbalance that can increase appetite, and partly because exhaustion can leave you with less determination to follow your goals.

High stress levels can also have similar effects, so working to reduce stress in your life can help your weight-maintenance goals. And as with weight loss, an important way to keep the stress down is to have good support for your goals.

Key Points

- Focusing on a healthy diet can help you on your journey towards better health and weight loss, but you must never forget that other factors are also important to include as a part of your lifestyle. Your diet, physical activity, and your biological make-up, all play a role in the way your body responds to the stresses of everyday life.

- Eating a variety of foods is the key for healthy life.
- One of the ways to eat healthy could be achieved by planning ahead, doing a food shopping list, cooking in bulk, and using leftovers for the following day.
- Nearly every process in your body requires water to function properly. Make sure you drink plenty of water, and always carry a water bottle with you.
- Avoid crash dieting. Instead, eat a well-balanced diet, which includes a variety of foods that provide your body with plenty of nutrients. Focus on healthy eating rather than dieting.

Chapter 3: Meals

"The core benefit of eating right is having the energy to meet your dreams and to live a fulfilling lifestyle."

Tony Robbins

How to Prepare Healthy Meals

If you are trying to change your eating habits for better health, weight loss, or to maintain your healthy weight, it is not just a matter of counting calories. It is far more important to take an overall view of how you eat, and that means developing good habits around food. Whether you are a busy person or not, you must remove all the barriers that prevent you from eating healthy.

Many fad diets recommend you to dramatically reduce the amount of food you eat or to cut out certain food types, but this is not a healthy approach. We need all the major food groups to function properly, although there are better and worse sources of them. A healthy diet is a well-balanced diet. Typically, a healthy meal should include:

- Vegetables, salads, and fruits – Around half your plate should be made up of these.
- Carbs should be unrefined, especially wholegrain versions of bread, pasta, and rice.
- Lean protein – This could be meat, fish, or eggs, but you can also get your protein from beans, legumes, or tofu.
- Fats in monounsaturated and polyunsaturated forms, such as olive oil, avocados, or nuts.
- Stick to water as your default drink, and drink plenty of it. The occasional tea (herbal teas are always fine), coffee, or alcoholic drink is okay, but avoid sugary drinks.

Once you have established what you need to eat for a healthy diet, take control of what goes into your meals. Where possible, cook from basic ingredients, and get used to checking labels for nutritional information if you need to buy anything pre-packaged.

If you are planning to eat out, you can research restaurants and find one that provides healthy food. You can also study the menu in advance online, and pick out a healthy option when you are not hungry. Most menus in restaurants have at least one healthy meal option that you can choose.

Of course, I do not think that I need to mention that you should avoid visiting fast food restaurants such as McDonalds, Burger King, or pizza delivery places, etc. Most fast food is high in sugar, salt, and trans fats, and is extremely processed. In addition to this, fast foods do not contain nutrients such as fibre or antioxidants, which are important for the health of your body.

Although counting calories is less important than some diets would have you believe, it is important to keep portions reasonably small. Perhaps you could use smaller plates, or half-fill your plate with vegetables or salad before adding anything else.

Eating regular meals is as important for healthy weight as food choices or portion sizes. Skipping meals is likely to make you eat more when you do eat, and it is harder for your body to process a large meal than a series of smaller ones. As much as possible, keep your meals at the same times each day, and try to avoid eating dinner too late in the evening.

Having regular snacks between meals can help you stick to your healthy eating — as long as they are healthy snacks, of course. Fruit, raw vegetables, and nuts are all good to nibble on. On the other hand, do not be too hard on yourself. Allowing yourself the occasional unhealthy treat can help beat the cravings, as long as you do not make too much of a habit of it.

In the rest of this chapter, you are going to learn how to implement your learning about healthy eating into practice, so that it can be accommodated into your busy life.

How to Make a Healthy Breakfast

You will often hear that breakfast is the most important meal of the day, but what does that really mean? Apart from that it is a bad idea to skip it, what you eat for breakfast is crucial in maintaining your healthy diet.

Why eat a healthy breakfast?

Sleep is an important phase in your nutritional cycle. While you are asleep, your body is processing the food you have been eating, stabilising your blood sugar, and detoxing your system.

This means that the first meal you eat after waking will set you up for the day, and more importantly, what you eat will set the tone for your day too. Eating a healthy, balanced breakfast (which should include drinking plenty of water) will boost your energy and brain power, as well as preventing you getting hungry before lunch, with the risk of grabbing unhealthy snacks. Apart from drinking water, a herbal tea is a good alternative. Some teas, such as fresh peppermint or ginger tea, contain antioxidants and vitamins, helping you fight disease and infections.

Many people start the day with a bowl of cereal, but that is not the healthiest breakfast. The problem is that the small bowl of cornflakes can have anything between six and eight spoons of sugar, and some people add more sugar to it. This kind of eating is extremely unhealthy and can cause you to eat more later on in the day, due to the drop in your blood sugar levels.

As with any meal, the two most important things are to ensure that you balance all the main food groups, and that each group is represented by healthy options. While portions should obviously not be too large, these are more crucial than cutting calories.

- Carbohydrates – It is vital to get the right carbs for breakfast, and that generally means either wholegrain cereal or porridge, containing little or no sugar. Alternatively, you could make your own healthy muffins or cakes with wholegrain or oatmeal ingredients.
- Proteins – Protein for breakfast does not have to mean a full English breakfast, but eggs provide a great source of breakfast protein, whether you like them boiled, poached, scrambled, or in omelettes. If eggs are off the menu, a great alternative is tofu scramble, which can be mixed with various vegetables for extra variety.
- Fruit and Vegetables – Besides combining vegetables, such as peppers, mushrooms, or onions, with tofu scrambles or omelettes, there is also the option of having a variety of fruit with your cereal or porridge. Blueberries, strawberries, and bananas, are perfect for this. Alternatively, you could combine your fruit with yoghurt or whip it up in a smoothie.
- Dairy – Greek yoghurt is a versatile breakfast ingredient, either eaten straight as a smoothie, or with fresh berries and some seeds. If your diet is dairy free, soya or coconut milk offer a fine alternative.

- Fat – Your breakfast should include some healthy fat, and using nuts or avocado will provide that. Having a scrambled egg and a couple of slices of avocado on a slice of wholemeal bread is a fantastic start to the day.

As with all healthy meals, though, the secret is to experiment. As long as you choose healthy options and cover all the food groups, your breakfast will set you up for the day. You should also make sure that what you choose is something you enjoy and like. Remember, healthy eating is not a chore; it is something you do for health, but also something you do because you like it too.

How to Make a Healthy Lunch

To some of my clients, the lunch is the most dangerous meal of the day. They are often away from home and in a hurry at lunchtime, and that makes it very easy to reach for an easily accessible, unhealthy, fast food option. How many times have you been to the shop during your lunch break, and bought something unhealthy such as a sandwich, a packet of crisps, a chocolate bar, and a bottle of Coke?

You see, with planning, it is not difficult to ensure that you have a healthy lunch. Planning things in advance will set you up for success. Many people have a habit of planning work-related stuff, but when it comes to their personal life, they fail to plan. Do not forget this: If you want to reach success in anything, planning is necessary.

Why is a healthy lunch important?

As lunch appears right in the middle of most people's time at work, it is important to top up your energy for the second half of the day. The right kind of breakfast will take you up to around 1 p.m., but you will need a boost around this time, to ensure that you make it to the end of the day with enough energy to continue being productive, and to avoid you moving towards unhealthy snacks.

The problem is that an unhealthy lunch can do the opposite. You will feel stuffed and sluggish, but it will not last. Before five o'clock, you will be tempted to reach for snacks, and the chances are they will be unhealthy too. This is not a healthy or productive picture to be a part of.

In order to avoid the temptation to grab something unhealthy, it is best to prepare your own lunch and take it to work with you. A good trick is to prepare it straight after dinner the night before; that way, you are making it while you are not hungry, so you are less likely to overdo it, and you are more likely to focus on health, rather than satiating your stomach's growls.

If you need to go to a café or restaurant for lunch (either because you have not brought any food or because you are going with friends or colleagues), then try to make sure you go somewhere that offers healthy options, and choose what you are going to order before you go in. This is especially important if you have company, as you can easily be swayed by what they are having. These days, we are able to check the menu online for any restaurant. This can help us make a decision whether we want to go there for a meal or not.

As with all meals, it is important to choose healthy options for all the main food groups. If you are taking your lunch with you, it helps to keep it simple.

Here are my recommendations for what to include in your healthy lunch:

- Your protein could, for example, come from chicken, tuna, tofu, or lentils.
- Having a wholemeal pasta or brown rice are versatile ways of ensuring you get good carbs in your lunch.
- Mix vegetables in with your wholemeal pasta or brown rice dish, or have a salad. You can also take some fruit with you — berries are always a good option: strawberries, blueberries, blackberries or raspberries. They are high in antioxidants and rich in fibre and vitamin C. They can lower your cholesterol and help the health of your heart. They can also support your weight loss, if that is your goal.
- Avocado or olive oil with your lunch will provide a healthy source of unsaturated fat.

And as always, make sure you drink plenty of water, rather than sugary drinks, keeping your tea, coffee, or alcohol to a minimum. A healthy lunch will keep your energy levels up till dinner without leaving you overfull.

How to Make a Healthy Dinner

After you have had a healthy breakfast to set you up for the day and a healthy lunch to give you a boost, it can be tempting to "reward" yourself with an unhealthy dinner. It is very common to feel this way and say, "I was eating healthy all day; therefore, I deserve to eat something unhealthy this evening." But this is not a smart idea.

Research shows that with each passing hour after breakfast, there is a decrease in the nutritious food we consume and we tend to eat less healthy foods at night in comparison to the rest of the day.

Let's look at why a healthy dinner is important.

Most people are familiar with the fact that eating an unhealthy dinner or eating late at night can affect their weight, but not everyone is aware that eating a healthy dinner can improve their health and sleep.

Dinner is the meal you take to bed with you. This means that its contents can have a strong effect on how well you sleep. An unhealthy dinner, for example, can result in your glucose levels falling while you sleep, and this can often wake you up. Similarly, failure to eat the foods that help create essential neurotransmitters, such as serotonin, can disrupt your sleep and leave you tired and depressed the following day, and perhaps even beyond.

Large, unhealthy dinners, and eating late at night can affect your digestion, which might keep you awake at night, as well as cause obesity and the risk of developing diabetes or cardiovascular disease.

Most of us have busy lifestyles these days, and it can be easy for dinner to get pushed back until late in the evening. This is not a good idea for several reasons. Besides the temptation to reach for something easy and unhealthy (such as calling at the takeaway on your way home from work), it means you are hungrier when you do come to eat. This can result in eating more than you need, and choosing unhealthy options because they seem easier, quicker, and more desirable to you at that moment.

Eating late also creates the problem that your body has less time to process the food before you go to bed. This leaves you badly prepared for enjoying a good night's sleep, and you are more likely to struggle to fall asleep, and probably wake up a few times during the night as a result. The next day, you are going to feel tired, sluggish, irritated, and probably quite low in mood.

The best approach is to plan your dinners in advance for the week, preferably when you have just eaten and are not hungry. This will result in you being sure to have the ingredients and to know what you are doing. Remember to include some quick recipes that you can reach for if you are rushed.

As always, make sure you include the main food groups in your dinners:

- Lean meat (especially chicken or turkey), oily fish, tofu, or beans will provide protein.
- Brown rice, wholegrain pasta, or quinoa for your carbs. Occasional boiled or jacket potatoes are OK, though consider sweet potatoes instead — they are a healthier option.
- Have salad as part of your meal, or else include vegetables such as spinach, broccoli, peppers, courgette, carrots, or legumes.
- Include avocado or have an olive oil based dressing on your salad. They are both good sources of fat.

If you want a glass of wine with your meal, or a coffee afterwards, make sure it is just one. In any case, as always, drink plenty of water with your dinner.

Get into the habit of serving your dinner on a small plate. This will make such a huge difference to the amount of food you eat. A tip that I often give to my clients is to serve their plate with salad or vegetables first, then add foods such as meat or fish, and then the rest of the food, which is usually carbohydrate-rich food, such as rice, pasta, or potatoes.

By arranging your plate in this particular order, you will notice that by the time you put all the veggies and meat or fish on your plate, you will have only a limited amount of space for anything else, which is often a carbohydrate-rich food. This is a great way of serving your evening meals as at this time of the day, your body requires less carbohydrates, as it needs less energy nearing the end of the day.

How to Snack Smart

I often hear people say that they have problems with choosing healthy snacks. Their main meals — breakfast, lunch, and dinner — are often okay, well planned and nutritious, but when it comes to snacking, they tend to eat mainly sugary foods, such as chocolate, biscuits, cake, or salty foods such as crisps. Does this sound familiar?

About 20 years ago I was someone who kept eating all the wrong foods, especially snacks. I used to binge on chocolates and other sugary-rich foods. But I also did lots of running at the time — at least five miles per day, six to seven days a week. This supported my weight loss, but I felt lethargic quite often, not understanding why.

Snacks are an important part of our diet. Used wisely, they can help keep our blood sugar levels steady between meals, which is beneficial not only for our overall health but also our performance at whatever we do during the day.

It would be much simpler if we could just stick to breakfast, lunch, and dinner, and eat nothing else. However, it does not work like that. There are good reasons for needing snacks at various points during the day, but these come with risks too.

In addition, and rather counter-intuitively, smart snacking can help you to avoid overeating. This is because it prevents you from getting too hungry at mealtimes, which could result in overestimating the portions you need.

On the other hand, many of the most popular snacks, the ones people tend to reach for without thinking, are packed with sugar or unhealthy trans fats. These can have the opposite effect, causing spikes in blood sugar that mess up your healthy eating patterns.

The key to smart snacking is doing it deliberately. Plan it. One of the main traditional problems with snacking is that we tend to reach for snacks automatically, and we are barely aware of what we are doing. This could be in any situation from being absorbed in work to sitting in front of the TV during the evening.

To snack smart, plan your snacks just as you plan your main meals. Choose in advance what will make a good snack, and either prepare it to take with you or know where you are going to get it from. Similarly, choose the times when snacks will be most beneficial, and not just when you have "the munchies."

Make sure you eat your snacks slowly and mindfully. That way, you will know exactly what you are putting into your body and be aware of when you have had enough.

As always, like with all other meals, concentrate on healthy options from the main food groups, but in forms that can be conveniently carried and eaten on the go. Also, make sure your snacks contain plenty of fibre, which has a role in controlling both cholesterol and blood sugar, as well as aiding digestion.

Some examples might be:

- Most kinds of fruit and berries
- Nuts, seeds, and chickpeas – This can include peanut butter
- Greek yoghurt – It goes well with fruits and some seeds or nuts
- Vegetables that can be made into easy snacks, either raw or roasted
- Avocado – perhaps in the form of guacamole
- Oatcake with nut butter – If you decide to have one from the jar instead of homemade one, it is important that you read a food label and make sure you do not consume one with a high level of sugar

Remember, smart snacking should still be a pleasure, not a chore, so choose snacks you are going to look forward to.

How to Make Healthy Food Swaps

When faced with changing your unhealthy diet to a healthy one, it may seem like a very hard thing to do. Some people might be tempted to give up, but it does not have to be complicated. By concentrating on one food at a time and making healthy swaps, you can transform what you are eating, and develop healthy habits in that area of your life.

Before you start diving straight in and swapping foods blindly, it is a good idea to keep a food journal for a few weeks, establishing what you are eating regularly, then list each food you eat regularly, marking the ones you feel you need to change. This can also help you to identify eating habits and to look at reasons why you might be lacking in energy at certain times of the day. It is likely that you are not even aware of the effect your meals are having on your energy levels, but a diary will show you that information quite clearly.

The next stage is to decide what you are going to put in its place. This will take a little research and soul-searching, but the best approach is to identify something with a high nutritional value that could easily take the place of the food you are abandoning, whether as a snack or as a meal ingredient. However, think about whether you are likely to enjoy it, as well as whether it is good for you. You have to enjoy the food you are eating; otherwise, you are simply going to abandon it for an unhealthy, yet more delicious option.

The swaps you make will depend on what you like to eat, but they should be based on a good balance between the main food groups. Here are just a few examples you might want to consider:

- Breakfast – Change your sugary cereal for overnight oats, with fruit in place of added sugar. Instead of a slice of white toast with butter, have an egg on wholemeal bread.
- Lunch – Instead of having a sandwich made of white bread, make it with wholegrain bread, or have a small jacket potato served with tuna and plenty of salad.
- Dinner – If pasta is your favourite meal, have home-made tomato-based sauces with your wholegrain pasta instead of creamy sauces.

- Snacks — Instead of chocolates or packets of crisps, have a few Brazil nuts or a handful of almonds. And instead of a bag of chocolate biscuits, why not have a couple of oatcakes with hummus or cut apple with peanut butter.
- Drinks — Instead of orange juice or a Coke, add slices of your favourite fruit to your water. This will give a nice taste to the water, and it will add lots of health benefits. Far from being bland, it is the most refreshing of all drinks.

Forcing yourself to eat foods you dislike because they are good for you could wear away your motivation. There is usually a perfectly acceptable alternative, as you can see in the examples I just mentioned.

Like with anything else, it is important to develop a good habit. A habit of eating healthy is like developing any other habit. The healthier you eat, the easier it will become, and after a while, you will notice that your body is asking for the healthy food alternative. I will never forget my first taste of avocado. I put it in my mouth and thought "I never tasted something so tasteless in my entire life," but now I can eat it every day.

When making food swaps, think of the healthier alternative, and you will be just fine. It does not need to be always super healthy, but healthier compared to what you usually have. Any effort in this regard is better than no effort.

To download your *"5 Day Healthy Meal Plan for Busy People,"* which is packed with easy and simple meal ideas, and to receive a special bonus, *"20 Items That You Must Have on Your Food Shopping List,"* go to www.bit.ly/bundle-fit-and-healthy.

How to Read Food Labels

In my book, *Get Your Sparkle Back: 10 Steps to Weight Loss and Overcoming Emotional Eating,* I wrote a section called "Understanding Food Labels." I would like to highlight the most important points from this section as it is important to learn how to read food labels in order to understand the nutritional values of the foods you eat. If you do not understand what you are supposed to look for when reading food labels, then you will never know what you are putting inside your body.

Here is the brief description of this section, and my top tips to help you gain a better understanding of food labels:

- Check the ingredients list – Most pre-packed food products have an ingredient list attached. They are always listed in order of weight, so the main ingredients in the packaged food always come first. Heavily processed foods can have over 30 ingredients. It is recommended to choose products with 5 ingredients or less.

- Calories – My advice is to keep an eye on calories, but do not get too obsessed with them. It is far more important to pay attention to the ingredient list rather than the amount of calories in the food. Calories can come from healthy or unhealthy food, and the focus always has to be on consuming healthy calories/food. For instance, whether 100 calories come from healthy or unhealthy foods, they always represent 100 calories, but the nutritional value that we receive from them is very different.
- Traffic-light colours – You will often find a colour-coded nutrition label on the front of packaging, with red, yellow, and green colours. This shows whether the food contains high, medium, or low amounts of fat, saturated fat, sugars, and salt.
- Learn where the sugar is – Sugar has many names. There are over 60 names for sugar. The only way to know where the sugar is hidden is to learn the most commonly used names for sugar.

Other information found on food labels show possible allergies and total carbohydrates, as well as nutritional claims, such as reduced fat, fat free, no added sugar, etc. Many of those nutritional claims are often misleading, and manufacturers try to hide controversial ingredients by naming them differently, trying to cover the truth from consumers. It is important to be aware of this when doing food shopping and reading the food labels of your favourite foods.

You should also know that there are over 3000 food additives added to foods. Some of them are known to have negative effects on your health. There is a large section on this topic in my book, *Get Your Sparkle Back: 10 Steps to Weight Loss and Overcoming Emotional Eating,* where you can learn more about this.

Understanding the meaning of food labels will help you make the right food choices.

My advice is to stick to eating whole foods. When eating whole and natural foods, you do not need to play a guessing game to try to find out what ingredients are hiding in those foods. Real foods do not have labels.

Key Points

- Do not skip breakfast, and always choose healthy options.
- Prepare lunch straight after dinner and take it with you to work the following day.
- Plan dinner in advance for the whole week.
- Eat your snacks slowly and mindfully, to make you aware when you have had enough.
- Try to remove all unhealthy foods from your kitchen, to avoid temptation.
- Always read food labels. It is important to learn the meaning of the information displayed on them such as traffic-light colours and nutritional claims.
- Go to www.bit.ly/bundle-fit-and-healthy to download your *"5 Day Healthy Meal Plan for Busy People"* and to receive a special bonus *"20 Items That You Must Have on Your Food Shopping List."*

Chapter 4: Exercise

"Yes, exercise is the catalyst. That is what makes everything happen: your digestion, your elimination, your sex life, your skin, hair, everything about you depends on circulation."

Jack LaLanne

How to Find Time for Exercise

Healthy eating is the key to health and weight loss, but it has to form part of a generally healthy lifestyle. Many people know that exercising, in addition to healthy eating, is essential for losing weight, but not many people are aware of the full benefits of exercise and how moving their body can support their health, mind, and well-being.

Studies show that physical exercise can benefit your health and psychological well-being, as well as speed up your metabolism and decrease the risk of stroke and heart disease.

I am aware that many people struggle with fitting regular exercise into a busy lifestyle and I do understand that for some people, finding time to exercise when living a busy life is the last thing they think of. If your idea of exercise is spending an hour or two in the gym every day, you might simply not have time. Fortunately, it does not have to be that difficult. The gym is not the only place where you can get some exercise and it is definitely not the only type of exercise that you can implement into your busy lifestyle.

On the whole, most people who do not exercise either do not want to, or believe they do not have time for it. Not much can be done if someone really does not want to exercise, but we can all relate to not having enough time. However, this is partly an excuse and partly misunderstanding what is really needed in an exercise regime.

We all find time to do the things we really want to, such as watching our favourite TV programmes. The good news is that the extra energy you will get from exercise will more than make up for the limited amount of time you need to put into it.

Fortunately, it is not actually necessary to set aside long stretches of time to get your exercise in. Research shows that short bursts of exercise can do you just as much good as extended periods – perhaps even more good.

Studies have suggested that multiple bursts of 10 minutes of exercise, called high-intensity interval training (HIIT), often produce better results than a continuous session of up to 40 minutes. The short-burst groups tended to end up doing more exercise over the course of a week, and therefore, lost more weight, not really realising that they had done as much exercise as they thought. This is ideal for those who are low on time but high on motivation.

In addition, it has been shown that short bursts of exercise can give health benefits that are equal to longer periods. This includes lowering cholesterol and decreasing the risk of heart disease, and HIIT training is shown to be a more enjoyable type of exercise in comparison to moderate intensity continuous training, mainly because participants were required to spend less time exercising.

There are many strategies for fitting in 10-minute bursts of exercise, depending on the needs of your lifestyle, but here are some of the most common:

- Get up 20 minutes early and go for a brisk walk or run before breakfast. Alternatively, you could do some yoga.
- Walk or cycle to work or to the shops, if possible. If it is too far, either park a little farther away, or else get off the train or bus at the stop before.
- Go for a walk during your lunch break, or if there is a gym nearby, you could have a short session there.
- If you have regular meetings at work, encourage your colleagues to turn them into walking meetings.

- Use stairs instead of the lift.
- Carry the shopping basket instead of pushing a trolley while doing the food shopping.

You can see now how exercising can easily become part of your everyday life. All you need to do is to want it enough.

How to Find the Right Exercise for You

One crucial part of a healthy lifestyle is to exercise. But what kind of exercise is the right one for you? Should you take up jogging or cycling, or should you join your local gym? Or maybe joining Pilates or Zumba classes would be a better idea?

The reality is that the right exercise depends on your particular needs, what you can fit into your lifestyle, and most importantly, what kind of exercise you enjoy. If you do not enjoy doing something, you will not stick to it. Therefore, do not think that doing something is a good idea simply because it sounds like a good idea. You need to enjoy what you do otherwise, you will not prioritise it over your job, business, family life, or other responsibilities.

In order to succeed, it is important to adopt exercise as an important part of your life, the same way you adopted your other habits, like taking the same route to go to work every day, or having a cup of tea or coffee every time you get home. This is another reason why you have to enjoy the exercise you do; it needs to be something you look forward to and want to do, not something you dread and procrastinate on. If you do that, it is simply not going to work, and you will end up abandoning it for something you deem to be more interesting or more important in that very moment.

It is also important to identify your needs. Exercise can be used to achieve a wide range of goals, from supporting your weight loss diet, maintaining your healthy weight, or achieving top fitness for a sport. Understanding your needs will help you to decide what you want to use the exercise for. You may be restricted by your general level of health; and in that case you should not try to push yourself further than your body allows, as it could cause serious damage.

Perhaps a chat with your doctor in that case could be a good route forwards. If you have back problems, for instance, speaking to your doctor will show you some exercise methods that are not going to aggravate your back issue, but will still allow you to grab the benefits of regular exercise. There is an exercise type for everyone; you simply need to explore your options a little in order to find it.

When looking for the right exercise make sure that it fits into your lifestyle; otherwise you will not pursue it when you are feeling tired or too busy. We do not all have the same amount of time or resources to devote to exercise. If you can afford to spend several hours a day and kit out a spare room at home with specialist equipment, then that is all well and good. The reality is that you will probably need to squeeze exercise periods into gaps in your schedule, and that is okay — whatever you can manage will benefit you.

It is important to realise that exercise can be part of your daily life. As discussed in the previous section of this book, you could walk or cycle at least part of the way to work, take the stairs instead of the lift, or leave your car at the far end of the carpark. There are many, many ways to include exercise into your everyday life. But the most important thing is that you do a type of exercise that you enjoy doing. For instance, in my case, I used to swim a lot and then went to the sauna to relax. I do not swim any-more; instead, I walk to the sauna and back. It takes me over an hour to do round trip. I understand that not everyone is able or free to walk for over an hour, but for this reason, it is important to find a type of exercise that fits your lifestyle and your abilities, and accommodate your needs.

Probably the most common reason why people fail to keep up their exercise regime is that it becomes a drag. We resist things we do not like doing, so it is important that you identify exercises you find fun, and stick to those as much as possible. If you hate weight training, for instance, it is not compulsory to do it. If you like running, but not when it is too cold or too hot out, or when it rains, you can have a plan B to run on a treadmill in a heated or air-conditioned gym on those days.

Create a habit of exercising. Some days you may need to force yourself to exercise. But when you start feeling the benefits of doing it, you will want to do it again and again. When exercise becomes your daily habit, your body will ask for it. The important thing to remember is that exercising should be enjoyable. Look at different options, and stick to those that you look forward to and find the most joy in doing.

How to Get Motivated to Exercise

Motivation is something that most people struggle with when it comes to exercise. Not everyone feels excited about running outside in the dark or the rain, or going to the gym and feeling pain in their muscles. Exercise is the type of activity that does not give us immediate satisfaction, but it can give us long-term benefits.

Let's discuss first the benefits of exercising. A number of studies have been done on this topic, and the findings show similar results — they all claim that regular exercise can improve health in many ways. Here are some of them:

- Exercise can increase your energy levels. Some people believe that exercise will make them tired, but the truth is that the exercise gives you more energy. This is due to the increased levels of endorphins. They are body's natural hormones and are released every time we do activity that requires a burst of energy. So, next time when you are feeling sleepy or tired, I suggest you go for a 15-minute brisk walk. You will feel more energised and much healthier.
- Exercise can help your brain health — A few studies suggest improved cognitive functioning after aerobic exercise.
- Exercise can help support weight loss — Most people are familiar with the fact that exercise can help them lose weight. Exercise speeds up your metabolism, which helps you lose weight. By doing exercise, you

are also building your muscles, which are responsible for faster calorie burning.

- Exercise can help you sleep better – It is shown that exercise can help you feel more relaxed. A number of studies suggest that exercise contributes to your quality of sleep. It will make you feel more energised during the day and help you sleep better at night despite the type of exercise you choose to do.
- Exercise can help you reduce the risk of chronic disease – It is been proven that regular exercise can help people to reduce the risk of type 2 diabetes, cardiovascular disease, insulin sensitivity, and many diseases related to obesity, such as visceral fat, better known as fat around the middle.

These are only a few benefits that you can gain from exercising. So, let's look at how you can start exercising on a regular basis. Here are some suggestions:

- Decide what your goal is – Do you want to gain muscle? Do you prefer to lose weight? Or is staying healthy your priority? Building muscle will require you to lift weights rather than do cardio exercises, as they are more suitable for supporting your weight loss. Decide what your goal is, and your goal will keep you motivated. Most importantly, find out why you want it. As I mentioned earlier, knowing why you are doing something is the vehicle to your destination. It creates desire and strength to move you towards your goal even when you are struggling or feeling depleted.
- Make a plan and write it down – This is such an important part of the process. It is much easier to be

disciplined when you create a plan. Write down in your diary times for exercising, how many times per week you will do it, what type of exercise you are going to do, etc. Writing it down will make a big difference to your life as this will increase the degree of your commitment. Things that are written down have such a big impact on us, as they represent the contract we made with ourselves.

- Be consistent – Consistency is the key. Consistency creates new behaviour, and new behaviour creates a new habit. Developing your exercise routine will give you the discipline needed for making exercise a part of your life. Establishing what your goal is, and writing down your plan, will help you with the consistency of doing your exercise.

Setting the right routine around your exercise is important and here are some suggestions on how to do it:

- Schedule your exercises.
- Stop making excuses.
- Make it as a social event.
- Get a habit of doing it, and then ask your friends to join you.

When routine is established, it gets easier. It is not a chore anymore, and it is something you automatically do without thinking about it. When you start seeing the results of your actions, you will want to keep repeating the action.

How to Move More

Humans originally evolved to be constantly on the move, but modern life is increasingly sedentary, which poses serious threats to our health. The truth is, you do not actually need to move much; you simply need to develop habits of movement, which force you to get your heart rate up, your muscles on the go, and give you the benefits of exercise, no matter how light.

In today's society, it is very easy to not move much. We sit in a car to get to wherever we are going. We spend a good deal of our working hours sitting down, and when we get home, we sit in front of the TV or the computer. The less we move, the less we want to move, and as a result, we simply do not move.

Lack of exercise is combining with today's unhealthy diet to create an obesity epidemic, but that is not the limit of the health problems of a sedentary lifestyle. Many studies show that a sedentary lifestyle is dangerous for our health. It is linked with an increase in type 2 diabetes, cardiovascular disease, and some types of cancer. It is bad for our mental health and can contribute to depression and anxiety. Sitting for too long can also slow down our metabolism, which will contribute to weight gain. It is a vicious circle in so many ways.

Many people do not exercise at all. Others do not even move very much. It is not enough to spend half an hour at the gym if you spend the rest of the day sitting down. While your time at the gym may be good for your overall health, exercise is far more effective if you do it little and often.

For instance, while watching TV, you could also be using a treadmill or stationary bike. While waiting for the kettle to boil, you can do a few squats. You can also do them while brushing your teeth. Imagine if you do a few minutes of exercise every morning and evening while you are brushing your teeth and during the day while waiting for the kettle to boil. If you are finding squats too difficult to manage, then walking in the same spot is an easier way to start moving your body. You will notice a significant difference to your fitness level after a while, simply by encouraging your body to move more, a few times a day every day. Remember, consistency is the key.

Do you ever spend any time waiting for a bus or train to arrive? Instead of sitting down at the bus stop and waiting for the bus, maybe you can stand up. Instead of standing in the same spot and waiting for the train, how about you spend that time walking up the platform? All those minutes would add up, and at the end of the week, you would have completed a decent number of minutes exercising. Can you see now how easy it is to find the time to move, to exercise, and to improve your health? It does not need to be hard or time consuming.

Try incorporating exercise into your life by taking one step at a time and make it a habit. If you have a sedentary job, it helps to plan it so that you can spend some of it on your feet, such as in walking meetings. If you work from home, consider investing in a standing desk. One of the most valuable solutions, though, is micro-breaking. This means that you take a brief break every 20 minutes or so to get up and move your body about – fidgeting with intent. It helps if you set up a timer or use an app to remind you when you need to take a break.

Of course, not all exercise needs to be formal. As I mentioned earlier, it can be as simple as sometimes leaving the car at home, parking on the far side of the car park at the supermarket, or taking the stairs instead of the lift.

The problem can be that exercising takes resolution, and it is easy to slip back into old habits. You need to create new habits that you will feel motivated to stick to. The best way of doing this is to make it fun. For instance, instead of jogging, how about dancing regularly? Or make sure you have your daily exercise by getting an energetic dog or playing with your kids.

You may not entirely get rid of the need for sitting down for a substantial portion of the day, but by building the habit of moving into your routine, you could find yourself generally healthier, more positive, and happier.

Key Points

- A sedentary lifestyle can negatively impact your health. Make exercising a habit, and include it in your daily or weekly routine.
- Studies show that multiple bursts of 10 minutes of exercise can give health benefits that are equal to longer exercise sessions.

- When searching for the right exercise, focus on your goals. Choose the exercise and plan your exercise regime according to your abilities and your needs, whether it is weight loss you want to accomplish, building muscles, or maintaining a healthy weight.
- Walking to the shop instead of driving, carrying the basket instead of pushing the trolley, walking up the stairs instead of taking a lift, and doing squats while waiting for the kettle to boil, can be all counted as part of your daily exercise. These little habits can improve your health and add years to your life.

Chapter 5: Lifestyle

"Looking good and feeling good go hand in hand. If you have a healthy lifestyle, your diet and nutrition are set, and you are working out, you are going to feel good."

Jason Statham

How to Find Time When You Do Not Have Time

"I don't have time" is a wonderful phrase.

Suddenly, you have the perfect excuse for everything you do not get around to doing, and for everything you did not achieve: "I'd love to, but I don't have time." Be honest with yourself: Is this a reason or an excuse?

When you say, "I don't have time," you are giving yourself permission not to do things. Whether it is exercising, losing weight or cooking a healthy dinner, it is often an excuse and not the real reason.

It looks very different if you say, "It's not a high-enough priority." This immediately puts it right back as your own responsibility, and you have to ask yourself honestly, "Do I really want this enough to find the time for it?" Everything you do on a daily basis is a matter of priority. If you want it enough, the time will be there, and your planning will encompass it; do not forget, planning is a habit. The more you do it, the more comfortable you will feel doing it.

When planning becomes part of your everyday routine, you will notice that many things you usually do can be reduced to take less time, which will free up extra time to be able to do things that you could not do before.

You can find time if you want to enough. It is simply a matter of priorities. Every minute of the day, all of us are putting our main priorities first. It is important that you decide what your priorities are and how you are benefiting from them.

The reality is that we often end up wasting time by not knowing what it is we want to achieve. Because of this, we fill in a lot of our time with whatever's to hand, such as checking our social media, and cannot fit in what we would really prefer to be doing. By being more mindful of your goals and the things you want to achieve in your life, no matter how big or how small, you will be able to find the time to make small steps towards achieving them. Any progress is good, whether it is small, large, fast, or slow.

The best way to keep yourself on track is to make an activity list at the start of the week. Planning ahead is crucial. This should include both the things you need to do and the things you want to do, assigning an appropriate amount of time for each activity. You can use any format that is convenient, but handwriting a list helps it stick in your memory, and also gives you a good point of reference to look back on when you need a boost of motivation. It is normal to have lapses in motivation as you go through a working week, after all.

Of course, your week is not always going to go according to plan, but if you have a schedule, it is a lot easier to readjust without forgetting what you really want to do. Planning helps you to focus, and gives the structure to the path ahead. Knowing the path you need to take will help you put your priorities in order of importance. This is hugely important when you feel overwhelmed with responsibilities and a lot is going on in your life. This will help you feel less stressed and also help you find some free time within your busy schedule.

Often, it is the stress of feeling short of time that makes that very lack of time worse, since it drains your energy. That means taking time out to feel good can give you back more time, and therefore increase your productivity levels in whatever you are focusing on.

This could be improving your health with exercise or healthy eating. It could be improving your mental state with yoga or meditation. It could be energising yourself with a hobby you love, or spending time with friends or family that stimulate you. It could simply be getting enough sleep. Whatever you need to do to feel good could help you find the extra time you need for your other activities.

How to Stop Procrastinating

We are all procrastinators at times. We delay completing certain tasks, and we put things off; instead of doing something today, we leave it for tomorrow. But why do we do it? How do we benefit from this behaviour? There must be a reason for behaving this way, is there?

Edward Young, an English poet living in the 18th century, said that procrastination is the thief of time. I agree with this statement. We start doing something, but do not finish it. We leave it for the next day, or the next week. Before you know it, a huge amount of time has passed and that task, the one which began as routine, is now hugely urgent. That causes stress and panic, two things that are extremely detrimental to your health and well-being.

We procrastinate for different reasons. Sometimes we procrastinate because we want to be perfect and want to do everything right, but we believe that we cannot do it the way we ought to do it. Sometimes we procrastinate doing tasks that are not pleasurable. At other times we are too scared of failure, and sometimes we are even scared of success, so we avoid doing things that we are supposed to be doing.

Whatever the reason is, we try to hide from our emotions by delaying the process, so that we do not need to feel a certain way. You could say that procrastination is there to keep us safe, to protect us from certain emotions, but on the other hand, procrastination can steal our joy and peace, bring anxiety, and make us worried. Feeling this way can make us feel drained and negative about life. It is far better to avoid procrastination as much as possible, to kick the negative effects out of your life.

Procrastination can cause lots of stress. This is especially bad if you have too much happening on an everyday basis. Procrastination is bad for your mental health and can affect your self-esteem and self-confidence, as well as introducing the feeling of guilt. Seeing everyone else progressing when you feel stuck and unable to move forward is not a nice feeling to have, and it is one that is likely to zap away your confidence and make you wonder why nothing you try ever goes the way you plan.

Put simply, when you procrastinate, you are leaving things to be done later. You are leaving things for another time, another day, another month. This will just add more frustration and stress to your already busy life, as you will not be achieving things that you want to achieve, or completing tasks that you need to complete. This will not help you feel less busy; it will actually add more business to your already busy life.

Be honest with yourself. Ask yourself how motivated you are to achieve the goals you are working towards. Without motivation, your energy will be low, and you will postpone jobs, both big and small, for another time. Procrastination will make you feel even busier in the end, not to mention far more stressed.

Here are some of the ways to deal with procrastination:

- Prioritise the most important things, and do them first thing in the morning. Piling up jobs to do later will cause more stress.
- Recognise what procrastination is trying to protect you from.
- Plan in advance so that you can make the time for things that need doing.
- Set time limits for your tasks, but do not be too hard on yourself if you go over by a couple of minutes.

How to Lead a Healthy Lifestyle When You Do Not Have Time

We all want to be healthy; who would not want that? The problem is that many people believe that their busy lifestyle does not allow them to find time for looking after their health. But healthy living does not have to mean spending hours in the gym or preparing insanely complex meals. All it takes is to make it important enough to you, and soon you will find that you have all the time you need for a healthy lifestyle.

Exercising when you do not have time is hard for many people, but exercise is not separate from the rest of your life, and you do not necessarily have to set aside a long stretch of time to do it. If you can manage an hour in the gym every day, that is fine; but otherwise, you can simply spend a few minutes doing simple stretches each time you stop for a break.

Similarly, healthy walking or cycling can be built into your daily routine. Even if you have a long daily commute, arranging it to include a 5-minute walk should not be too difficult. Could you perhaps walk down to the local shops in less than the time it would take you to drive to the supermarket?

Something that I often suggest my clients do is to stand up or walk while you are talking on the phone. I have noticed that people often sit down in order to speak on the phone, but actually, if you spend that time walking around, it adds up to the number of steps you do daily. Remember: one step at a time.

Being busy or lacking time should never be a reason for eating unhealthy, certainly when it comes to snacks. Many healthy snacks, such as fruit, nuts, or vegetable sticks, for instance, take no longer to prepare than grabbing a chocolate bar or a bag of crisps. You just need to be organised so that you have healthy snacks on hand when you need them.

One of the ways to deal with this is to always carry healthy snacks with you, such as have a bag of nuts or seeds in your handbag, or have a banana in your gym bag, or have a healthy protein bar in your car, or have a bag of oatmeal cakes in your desk in the office. Knowing that you have something healthy on hand will stop you from buying a chocolate bar or ice cream while paying for the petrol or catching a morning train to work.

Many people complain about lack of time when it comes to preparing meals. My experience is that preparing a healthy meal does not need to take longer than ordering a pizza or heating up a ready meal from the supermarket. Keep a folder of healthy and quick recipes to call on when you need them or simply go on the internet and type "quick and healthy recipes" — you will find lots of them there. Alternatively, you can have your own healthy ready meals available by preparing and freezing them when you do have time. Of course, drinking plenty of water takes no extra time at all.

Getting enough good quality sleep is a must. Ensuring that you have around eight hours sleep each night is likely to give you that time back. You will be more energised during the day and get through your schedule more quickly. Similarly, periodically taking five or ten minutes to meditate will improve your performance.

Healthy living is about the mind and emotions too, and it is important to have a social life that will boost your mental state. You do not need extra time for this; however, simply save your social time for people and activities that will help, not hinder, your aim of healthy living.

How to Create the Lifestyle That Is Right for You

No single factor can be named responsible for living a healthy life or having a slim body. There is no one-size-fits-all prescription for the right lifestyle, since it depends largely on your preferences, but there are certain general things to bear in mind. I will name four of them.

Get Plenty of Sleep

In today's round-the-clock world, it can be easy to skimp on sleep. This is bad for your general health and weight loss, since sleep is important for processing nutrients and detoxifying, as well as production of hormones that affect your satiety and hunger levels.

I suggest you find the routine that gives you the best night's sleep. I already covered this in Chapter One of the book, and I suggest you go back to this section, and if you have not already done so, start practising some of the habits that I suggested there.

I want to highlight that quality of sleep is one of the most important factors for your physical and mental health, and the power of good sleep should never be underestimated.

Make Physical Activity Fun

Some people just love weight training or pounding the treadmill, and that is great. If you find this a chore, however, it can be difficult to find the motivation to keep it up.

While you may still want to do some intensive training, it can be valuable to take up something active that you find fun, especially if it also offers a social aspect.

Taking up dancing or a sport can answer your needs, or why not join a club (or even a group of friends) to walk or cycle in the countryside? The important thing is that it is something you will thoroughly enjoy, while getting fit.

Make Your Social Life Positive for Health

Doing a hobby that you enjoy can help your mental and physical health in many ways. If you like walking, why not join a walking club? If you like reading, why not join a book club? If you like playing tennis, why not join a tennis club? Doing what you love, and being surrounded by like-minded people who love the same thing as you, can bring lots of enjoyment. When doing something gives you pleasure and makes you feel good, you will find time for it even if you live a busy lifestyle.

Make Your Social Life Positive for Weight Loss

Obesity is becoming an epidemic in the Western world, and maintaining a healthy weight needs to be your focus. All too often, people fail in their weight loss goals because their social life actively fights against them. After all, so many social gatherings traditionally revolve around unhealthy food or alcohol, and you may feel under pressure to conform.

This does not mean you need to cut yourself off from your friends. Instead, you could take the initiative and start suggesting social activities that do not revolve around food and drink, and if they involve physical activity, even better.

The most important thing to remember is that you did not decide to lose weight in order to punish yourself. You made the decision so that you could enjoy life more. Creating a lifestyle you can enjoy that still supports your goals will make it far more likely that you will succeed.

How to Make Your Surroundings Work for You

We are all profoundly influenced by what surrounds us and who surrounds us. Therefore, it makes sense to ensure that your surroundings work for you, not against you, by taking control of your environment and choosing people you want to spend time with.

One of the biggest enemies of staying on the right track of eating healthy is not preparing yourself in advance. I know I keep repeating myself, but I cannot stress enough the importance of planning things in advance. When it comes to weight loss, for instance, craving the foods you used to enjoy could be enemy number one. While the way to beat this is through positive thinking, removing temptation can also be valuable. Both in your home and your workplace, make sure, as much as possible, that you have only healthy food and snacks available. This can only be achieved with careful planning.

Of course, your workplace may not be 100% under your control, and management may not be willing to remove vending machines containing chocolate bars, crisps, and sugar-laden drinks. However, you can make sure you have plenty of healthy snacks at your desk so that you have no reason to use those machines.

It is also vital to surround yourself with people who are going to support you, whatever you choose to do. Whether friends, family, or work colleagues, you need people who are happy to eat, drink, and live healthy while you are around, rather than constantly trying to derail your efforts.

Create an environment that encourages exercise. It is easy to get lazy if your environment is set up to discourage exercise. For example, if everything you need is within arm's reach of your sofa at home or your desk at work, there is no incentive to get up and move around. Forcing yourself to get up and move around, including going up and down the stairs, will help keep you fit.

In the same way, you need to be surrounded by people who will encourage you to exercise. Try to gravitate towards friends who will go on walks or bike rides with you, rather than those who encourage sedentary pastimes. That does not mean you have to cut these people off as friends, but do not depend on them for inspiration.

On your days off, choose to go for a walk instead of watching TV or going to the cinema, and find a friend who likes to do the same thing. It is much easier to be motivated when you do things with someone who has a similar outlook on life as you do.

It is also important to make your environment positive in order to succeed. You will find it a lot easier to achieve your health or weight loss goals if you are in an environment that encourages positive feelings. This includes, of course, surrounding yourself with people whose positivity rubs off on you, but the strategy of decluttering your home also applies to this. Living in a cluttered home can weigh you down. My suggestion is to get rid of anything you do not really need. That includes things that you possess, as well as people in your life whose energy weighs you down.

Jim Rohn, a motivational speaker, once said, "Who you spend time with is who you become." If you are spending most of your time with negative people or people who do not prioritise healthy lifestyles over their old and unhealthy habits, then you are most likely to follow their steps and not progress to the next level. But if you make sure you surround yourself with positive people, who have adopted a healthy lifestyle, then your direction in life will be much more positive.

Everything we do in life is a matter of choice. We cannot choose family or work colleagues, but we are in the position to choose friends. And the quality of life you want to live is your responsibility, whether you are a busy person or not.

Key Points

- Exercise should be seen as a reward to your body, not a punishment.
- Make an activity list at the beginning of each week, so that you are well prepared, both mentally and physically, for your exercise days.
- Have homemade healthy ready meals available by preparing and freezing them, so that you can have them when you are too busy.
- Make your environment positive. Get rid of things and people that pull you down and work towards creating an environment that lifts you up and supports your goals.

Chapter 6: Self-Care

"Self-care is so much more than a beauty regime or an external thing you do. It has to start within your heart to know what you need to navigate your life."

Carrie-Anne Moss

How to Take Care of Yourself When You Do Not Have Time

You know you need to take care of yourself, whether that means exercising, eating well, doing yoga, meditating, or spending quality time by yourself or with your family or friends, or enjoying your favourite hobby such as dancing, painting, or reading. The trouble is you have so much to fit into so little time. As a result, you simply do not do it because you place higher importance on everything else.

Have you ever thought that not finding time for yourself could be just an excuse? Most people always manage to find the time for the things that are important, but the problem is that people do not find it important enough to do things for themselves. I see this happening all the time, and it is an extremely damaging habit to have.

Most of my clients often put other people's needs before their own. I understand that sometimes this is necessary and it has to be done, but by concentrating on other people rather than on yourself, you will always struggle with the lack of time, not to mention lower self-esteem and confidence. Here are a few strategies to help you.

Be Clear What You Want to Do and Why

Most of us have a tendency to waste emotional energy on what we are failing to do, instead of concentrating on what we want to do. It is important to be realistic, though. Set small, achievable goals, and if possible, schedule them in any time you are currently wasting. It is also important to realise that you cannot do it all; you are only human.

When you start scheduling your daily activities, whether they are personal or professional, you will notice that you suddenly have more free time. There are situations and emergencies that happen in people's lives that require immediate attention, and we need to act on it straight away, but we are often familiar with the tasks for the following day, or even the following week. Scheduling tasks and responsibilities that we need to accomplish will leave us with some free time for other things to do.

Similarly, be very clear about why you are doing these activities. "Because it's good for me" is not enough, and "because someone told me to" is even worse. Think about what you will gain and how great you will feel. At the same time, think about the cost of not doing it. When you think about how it will feel to procrastinate and put a task off, that can often be enough to force you to simply get on and finish it, to avoid the thought becoming a rather unwelcome reality.

Planning and Accountability Are Key

If you have simply decided to include something in your busy lifestyle, whether it is exercise, a hobby, or time with your friends, your decision can easily get lost in the rush. You are far more likely to succeed in fitting in the activity if you create some kind of structure, as this is an intention from your side.

For example, as well as practicing yoga in your own time, you could join a class that you have given a commitment to attend. Similarly, you could join a club to encourage you to pursue your hobby, or even just schedule reminders on your phone. Besides reminding you of what you intended, this will make you accountable. Even setting reminders for yourself is a personal accountability, while activities where other people are expecting you, are likely to take on a higher priority.

Enjoy the Moment

Even if you are being good to yourself, you will not get the full effect unless you are entirely there. So, focus 100% on where you are and what you are doing. Always be present and in the moment. Mindfulness is a good practice to try here, as this will help you to stay in the moment and not be thinking back over the past, or jumping into the future.

For example, if you are having time with the kids, try not to constantly check your phone for messages. If you are doing a yoga session, try not to let your mind drift off to a problem you are struggling with at work. Those concerns have their time and place, but you will not be taking care of yourself unless you give yourself the space to fully savour whatever special activity you have chosen to do right now. You are also stealing the joy away from yourself by doing this.

How to Make Yourself a Priority

We all have demands on our time from other people, especially if you are the primary caregiver for children, or if you are a carer for someone sick or disabled. In any case, though, the chances are that there will be demands from work, family, or friends, and that leaves you without much time for yourself. This is one of the reasons why so many people fail to prioritise themselves. Another reason could be a lack of self-respect. Some people hold the belief that other people deserve more, so they put their needs before their own.

We are taught from childhood to think of others, and this is largely right. Living a totally selfish and self-centred life is ultimately self-defeating. But everything has to be in moderation, and ignoring your own needs does not help anyone in the long run. Some people believe that prioritising their own needs is a selfish act. In reality, it is an act of self-care. When prioritising your own needs, you are giving yourself permission to be there for yourself. Your health, relationships, and happiness can benefit from learning how to prioritise your own needs.

Ultimately, it is only possible to help others if you are happy, healthy, and full of energy. If you are trying to look after your children, for instance, while feeling tired, drained, and frustrated, the chances are you will do more harm than good. This also applies to other areas in your life, especially your work. You have to look after yourself in order to give. You have to become your own priority.

How to look after yourself will depend on your needs, interests, and lifestyle, but general points include:

- Learn to say no. Trying to take on everything will only leave you exhausted, and you will end up doing everything poorly. It is perfectly fine to say no on occasion, and you should not feel guilty about it.
- Identify activities that drain your energy, and cut them out. If this is not completely possible, at least reduce them to a minimum
- Schedule some "me time" every day, and make it one of your highest priorities. Find a time when you are unlikely to be interrupted, even if this means getting up early or staying up late; however, do not go without sleep.
- Take regular time out, such as going out for the evening to do something you love. Even if you can only manage this once a week, make it a priority.

- Pay attention to your health, and prioritise anything you need to do to maintain it. Learning to nourish your body is the key.

The best way to ensure that you do not lose sight of your personal needs is to plan your day. Each evening, take a few minutes to list the things you want to do tomorrow, and put them into three groups: things you must do, things you ought to do, and things you would like to do if possible. Make sure the first group includes at least one (preferably more) "me thing," and make sure you tick it off the list as a priority.

As much as possible, specify when you are going to do each activity, but the idea is not to micromanage yourself. The purpose of your schedule is to ensure that you do not lose sight of the crucial things you need in order to take care of yourself, and ultimately of others.

How to Reward Yourself

Some people struggle to appreciate their own efforts, and often feel unable to give themselves a pat on the back for what they achieved, due to the lack of recognition of their own worth.

We are now going to look at how you can pay more attention to your needs and how to reward yourself simply for being who you are. In theory, losing weight and becoming healthier are their own reward. However, that is not how human beings are — we are conditioned to respond to more identifiable rewards. Rewarding yourself for your achievements, however small they are, is very much a part of self-care.

To give yourself a break when you need it most is so important, and it must be very high on your priority list. If you are a busy person most of the time, taking a break can be all the reward you need. It can be as simple as having a nap or taking a long, luxurious bath, or meditating for five to ten minutes, or reading a book somewhere quiet, in your garden or the bedroom perhaps, while being far away from other people.

Most of us have busy lives, and sometimes we struggle with it. Therefore, it is important to give yourself what you need. This must not be seen as selfishness, but necessity. Learning to be on your own and enjoying being by yourself will help you to get to know yourself better and provide you with energy, so that you can spend quality time with others.

The perfect way to emphasise what you are rewarding yourself for is to make your reward related to your achievement. For example, if you are rewarding yourself for reaching a landmark in your exercise regime, you could give yourself a new exercise outfit or a special water bottle. If you wanted to mark something more significant, you could splash out on a gym membership, or even a bike.

If you are celebrating reaching a milestone in your healthy-eating, weight loss program, there are food-related rewards that will not damage your efforts. You could buy a new cookery book, or you could simply treat yourself to a meal out in a healthy restaurant. Or, how about booking a spa day and enjoying a day of taking care of yourself? Book a facial treatment, pedicure, or a massage. Make your rewards healthy. They do not need to be always related to eating lots of foods or drinking a lot.

The activity you choose to do will depend entirely on your tastes, of course. Perhaps you love to go to concerts, the theatre, or the cinema. Your tastes could be anything from a museum or gallery to a sports event. Or perhaps you have a special interest — it does not matter what it is, as long as it is a reward to you. Use your imagination. Be creative.

Treating yourself to something specific, whether large or small, reminds you of the value of your achievement. That feeds into your sense of self-worth. Do not forget that the self-worth is what often rules your life. The more you value yourself, the more fulfilled you are going to feel.

How to Stress Less and Relax More

Stress is one of the main killers in today's society, and can make you turn towards unhealthy behaviours. One of them is to indulge yourself with junk foods. Familiarising yourself with your stressors will help you find the ways to reduce your stress levels. If you can identify what is causing you stress, it will be crucially important to your well-being.

It is all very well to aim towards getting fit and healthy and losing weight, but you are unlikely to achieve any of these goals if you are stressed all the time. When you are under stress, your body releases adrenalin and cortisol, two stress hormones that affect your mood, appetite, and happiness.

Reducing your stress levels and getting plenty of relaxation is key to many of your health goals. But how do you achieve this?

Identifying what is causing your stress is the number one step you need to take to tackle your stress level. In order to understand your stress, you need to understand your triggers. Knowing what your stressors are will help you gain control so that you will be able to manage your life better.

It is not always possible to avoid stress in every situation you face, but finding the main cause of your stress can help you deal with it better, or may even stop you from walking into situations that stress you out.

Scheduling tasks and everyday responsibilities is a popular way to reduce stress. Creating your own de-stress plan can help you at times when you feel like everything is on top of you and you feel like your life is out of balance. It might seem odd to say that imposing a schedule on yourself can help reduce your stress, but it can be a very powerful tool. Of course, it has to be the right schedule — one that incorporates all the activities that are most important to you, not just the tasks you are obliged to do.

The reason this can reduce your stress is that you are not constantly panicking and wondering how you are going to fit everything into your packed day. Your schedule allows you to approach each part of the day calmly, and even if life throws you a curveball, you will have a framework to fit in the new challenge. Do not forget that healthy diet and exercise play a massive role in deciding how your body will react to the stresses of everyday life. Having a healthy body can help you have a more relaxed attitude to life and create a healthier mindset.

One of the most important items to put into your schedule is to practise daily relaxation. I cannot stress enough the importance of including relaxation in your daily routine, even if it is only a few minutes here and there. This might include listening to your favourite music, walking, meditation, or other relaxation exercises — the important thing is that it is something that works for you and that you feel comfortable with. Many people benefit from implementing yoga in their morning or evening routine, while others benefit from having a warm bath and reading a book before bedtime.

Even if you are an extremely busy person, going for a walk to the local park or sitting in a coffee shop during your lunch break and reading a book, is something that can easily be done. If you cannot manage it every day, make an effort to do it some days. This will not only relax you, but it will help you be more productive when you return back to work after the lunch break.

In theory, you can practise relaxation at any time, but it is best to stick to the same time of day, as much as possible. This is partly because you are less likely to miss it if you have it scheduled in, but also because your mind and body will become accustomed to relaxing at that time and will be prepared for it.

Relaxation is not something to do as long as nothing more important comes up. That phone call or email will wait until you have finished what is genuinely important. And what is more important than your well-being?

How to Make Your Life More Fulfilling

Having a fulfilling life is a process and not a destination. It is about thriving and feeling proud of your actions so that you can achieve what you have set your heart on. Achieving the goal of leading a healthy lifestyle or achieving your weight loss goal is not all about healthy eating and exercises; it is also about being comfortable as yourself, in your own skin and for everything you are. Embrace it.

Sometimes the feeling of not being fulfilled leads to being busy. Also, ultimately one of the biggest causes of failing to achieve weight loss goals is feeling unhappy and unfulfilled. If you do not like yourself or your life, how can you believe you are worth the commitment to achieve happiness? If you do not even like yourself, how can you take care of yourself lovingly and with compassion? If you do not even like yourself, you will never feel fulfilled. Focusing on your happiness as much as the other well-known routes towards health and well-being, will push you further towards your goal.
So, how do you make your life more fulfilling?

There are certainly many ways that you can do this, but I will discuss three of the most important in my opinion.

Enjoy Being Yourself

When did you last make a decision to focus on yourself, here and now, and really mean it? Most of the time, we are so wrapped up in the future or the past, or things happening elsewhere, that we do not take the time to smell the roses and enjoy the here and now. Unless we live in the present, we do not even live, but we think we do.

We are being bombarded all the time with the idea that we need to be something else, or need to be someone else, or need to do something that we are not doing. There is nothing wrong with having aspirations and ambitions, but this can often leave us discontented with where we are now, and more importantly, with who we are.

One of the most valuable steps you can take to make your life more fulfilling is to appreciate and feel grateful for what you have and who you are. Do not compare yourself to others. You are not them. You are unique and special in your own way. Appreciate your uniqueness. Trying to be a different person is a rejection of yourself, and that can only lead to unhappiness.

The fact that you are unique is something to enjoy and embrace. There is nobody else like you, and that means you are special in your own skin. Ironically, understanding this is key to creating a healthy and happy mindset, which will power you on towards your other health-related goals.

Focus on Positive Relationships

We all need other people in our lives, and we want to feel needed. This is simply part and parcel of being a human being.

We need relationships with others, whether they are with family members, friends, or work colleagues, but relationships can be a double-edged sword. If you focus on people with negative outlooks or negative effects on you, they can easily drag you down. If you have ever heard the term "mood hooverer" or "energy vampire," this is someone who by simply being around makes you feel drained and negative about yourself. Avoiding these types of people is a good first step to take.

Try to be around people who give off the kind of vibes that energise you. If you need to be with negative people (family members or work colleagues, for instance), learn to understand what they are doing and why, and do not let them get to you. Give yourself regular breaks away from them, and manage the time you do spend with them to shield yourself against absorbing their negative vibes.

Positive relationships give meaning to our lives. They keep us healthy and happy. They help us be more positive, creative, and kind. They keep our spirit alive and increase our overall happiness and contentment. Being around people who make you smile and make you feel naturally uplifted can make a small outing, or a quick coffee something far more special than it is in reality, and therefore bring greater meaning to your life.

Be Clear About Your Goals and Ambitions

Yes, you should live in the moment, but that does not mean floating aimlessly. It is important to know what you want to achieve, and to set realistic goals to reach those achievements. If you do not do this, you risk wasting precious time and possibly having to live with regrets later in life.

The trick is to know where you are going and to enjoy the journey. Whether the important thing for you is your career, an artistic or sporting success, building a relationship, or reaching your target weight, you are most likely to enjoy it (and most likely to achieve it as well) if you value every step along the way.

This Is Not the End

This is not the end of your health journey; it is just the beginning. It is the beginning of your new habits, new behaviours, new lifestyle, and new you. I congratulate you for reaching for this book. It is an excellent start and a great first step. Give yourself a pat on the back. It is important that you recognise your efforts, and it is crucial that you understand your worth — because you are significant. Every single person is.

The path towards health, happiness, and contentment really does start with just one step, and you have shown a big commitment to take that step and move towards a brighter future.

There is no downside to focusing on your health and well-being. Everything in your life will improve quickly when you place focus on this. Not only will you feel better in yourself, have your health benefited, and have more time, but you will notice that the relationships in your life are improved too. When you are happy, positive, and healthy, you are almost magnetic, and people want to spend time with you. You are also more likely to attract the people into your life who are also exuding the same positive energy. As a result, life simply improves and gets better in ways you probably never imagined.

The increased confidence, which is a very welcome side effect of focusing on health and well-being, will also allow you to create opportunities without really trying. This could bring new energy into your life — perhaps a new career, a new relationship — it really could be anything!

Focusing on positive energy, health, well-being, and placing self-care as a priority, is the fast track towards a happy and more fulfilling existence. You have started your journey by reading this book and showing an interest in doing that for yourself. Keep going with your progress, and remember to reward yourself on a regular basis. Your health is in your hands.

Be kind to yourself and take care!

Lots of love XX

Silvana

Key Points

- Set small and achievable goals, and be clear about why you are doing it.
- Focusing on the present moment will bring more enjoyment into your life.
- Pay attention to your needs. Self-care is not only important to satisfy your own needs, but to be able to give to others the best of you.
- Reward yourself for your achievements, and make your rewards healthy.
- Practise daily relaxation such as yoga or meditation.
- Learn to enjoy being who you are.

GET FIT AND HEALTHY IN YOUR OWN HOME IN 20 MINUTES OR LESS

An Essential Daily Exercise Plan and Simple Meal Ideas to Lose Weight and Get the Body You Want

By Silvana Siskov

Thank you for purchasing
Get Fit and Healthy in Your Own Home in 20 Minutes or Less:
An Essential Daily Exercise Plan and Simple Meal Ideas to Lose Weight and Get the Body You Want

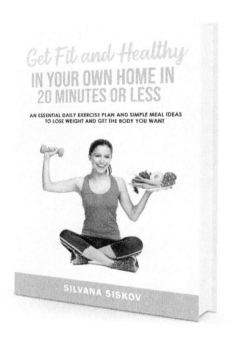

Go to www.bit.ly/bundle-fit-and-healthy
to download
"Get Slim and Healthy in 20 Minutes or Less Recipe Book,"
packed with delicious, simple and easy recipes,
to help you with your health and weight loss goals.

Introduction

Two of the most common resolutions people make are to eat more healthily and to exercise more, usually in an effort to lose weight. These are also the two resolutions that people break most often, simply because they find them too hard to maintain.

They do not have to be that hard, however, keeping fit and maintaining a healthy diet, are often seen by the vast majority of people as a sacrifice, instead of a part of their self-care plan. Therefore, the resolution to eat and exercise regularly is easily broken.

If you have ever been in this situation, perhaps you have not approached it in the best way. For example, you may have assumed that keeping fit involves at least an hour at the gym or a five-mile run every day. While you can certainly do either of these, it does not have to be like this.

If you are trying to fit an exercise regime into a busy lifestyle, you can do it in the comfort of your own home. Just 20 minutes a day will make a massive difference to your fitness levels, and you can even split that into two sessions of ten minutes each.

Similarly, healthy eating does not have to mean spending hours in the kitchen, preparing hard to obtain ingredients. You can easily make a wide range of healthy meals from a simple ingredients list, in as little as 20 minutes or less. This book will show you how to do this.

Eating well does not mean a limited range of bland recipes. The options are vast, and after you have been eating healthily for a while, you will wonder what you ever saw in fast food. Fad diets suck the energy out of you because your body is lacking essential nutrients. Eating healthy is different. It is the foundation for a good life. It is the choice that you make and it is something that you have full control of.

In the first two chapters of this book, you will learn the importance of both exercise and diet; the benefits of exercising and eating a healthy diet. You will be introduced to a variety of physical activities and healthy foods that can keep you in good health and support you on your journey to a healthy weight. You will also be shown how you can meet your goals in just 20 minutes or less.

In the next chapter, I will explain in more detail the kind of exercises you can do in the comfort of your own home. You will learn about warm-up exercises, how to exercise both your upper and lower body and how to get the most out of your stretching exercises.

Following that, you will receive some specific advice and plenty of simple ideas on how to prepare meals that are quick, healthy and delicious. Besides breakfast, lunch and dinner, we are going to look at how you can snack healthily throughout the day, as well as the best drinks to keep you fit and hydrated.

Finally, I will be giving you some advice on how to establish a routine that will allow you to stick to your healthy new lifestyle without it being a chore.

Getting fit and healthy does not have to be hard. You can do it in your own home in just 20 minutes or less; as long as you take the right approach.

In addition to all the great tips and meal ideas in this book, I am also offering you a free recipe book *Get Fit and Healthy in 20 Minutes or Less*. Go to www.bit.ly/bundle-fit-and-healthy and download your copy for free. You will receive a 29-page book, packed with healthy, simple and quick to prepare recipes. These recipes are designed to help you establish healthy habits, restore your energy levels and support your weight loss. The recipes are delicious and easy to prepare. The preparation time for each meal is only 20 minutes or less.

You will learn that healthy eating does not need to be difficult, expensive, time-consuming or tasteless. You will discover that with a little effort, you can achieve a healthy and fit body that you will feel proud of.

Chapter 1: Exercise

"Those who think they have no time for bodily exercise will sooner or later have to find time for illness."

Edward Stanley

Benefits of Exercising

Throughout most of human history, there was no need to build exercise into the daily routine, since people tended to live active lifestyles. Today, however, most of us travel by car, use labour-saving devices and sit down for most of our work and leisure activities.

That means that, whether we hit the gym or simply leave the car behind sometimes, it is vital to exercise consciously in a way that was unnecessary for our ancestors.

Exercising for Physical Health

According to the advice of the National Health Service (NHS) in the UK, "Whatever your age, there is strong scientific evidence that being physically active can help you lead a healthier and happier life." 150 minutes a week of moderate to vigorous-intensity activity has been shown to reduce the risk of many diseases. At the same time, extra exercise, such as playing sports or using the gym, intensifies this effect.

Exercises such as brisk walking, jogging, or cycling, for example, can reduce blood pressure and blood fat levels, as well as improve insulin sensitivity, body composition and cardiovascular fitness. These effects reduce the likelihood of developing the following conditions:

- Coronary heart disease and strokes (by 35%)
- Type 2 diabetes (by 50%)
- Various types of cancer (by 50%)
- Osteoarthritis (by 83%)
- Early death (by 30%)

This shows that including regular exercise into your life is a matter of priority and it is something that you must not ignore. Your health and the quality of your life greatly depend on it.

Exercising for Mental Health

Studies show that regular exercise can improve the brain's ability to handle stress and anxiety, as well as increasing the production of endorphins, which make you feel more positive. The overall effect is reduced stress and this seems to work even with a minimal amount of activity.

Regular exercise can also promote the growth of brain cells, especially in the hippocampus, the part of the brain that regulates memory and learning. It can not only improve general mental function as you grow older but may also reduce your risk of developing Alzheimer's disease.

Exercising for a Healthier Lifestyle

Besides fighting disease and promoting mental health, exercise can have a significant impact on your lifestyle. Of course, being healthier and feeling more positive can help you enjoy life more.

I love spending weekends going hiking. I do it whenever I can. It is such a pleasurable experience spending a day outdoors, enjoying the fresh air and being surrounded by the beauty of nature. I have adopted this activity as part of my life now and I love it.

I would like to encourage you to find an exercise you enjoy and then implement it into your routine. When it becomes routine, then it is something you do regularly. It becomes your lifestyle. You do not ask questions; you simply do it.

Exercise can also help you reduce weight, especially when you combine it with a healthy diet. It has also been proven to help with improving sleep, which underpins almost all aspects of a healthy lifestyle. We are all able to see the benefits of exercise for better sleep in children as those who have been running around all day crash out and have a good night's sleep. In contrast, those who spend all day sitting and playing with their electronic devices often experience problems sleeping. The effect is similar, regardless of age.

Regular exercise can help you feel more energised, improve your mood and even boost your sex drive, allowing you to enjoy a fuller and more satisfying sex life. You can receive all these benefits from an activity that is not only easy to do but which you also enjoy.

What Is the Best Type of Exercise?

So, we have established that exercising has numerous benefits, but what kind of exercise should you be doing? Assuming you are aiming to maintain a healthy body and perhaps support your weight-loss diet, rather than hitting peak fitness for the Olympics or winning a body-building prize, there are various approaches.

A wide range of exercises can meet your needs, as long as you use them regularly. Ultimately, the best type of exercise is the one that you enjoy and feel comfortable doing. You will not notice the benefits of exercising if you do not like doing it or if you only do it once in a while. It is something that you need to implement regularly, so eventually exercise can become a part of your routine. We will talk more about this in the last chapter of this book which focuses on how to establish a healthy daily routine.

Now, let us look at the different types of physical activities that you can engage with.

Moderate Aerobic Activity

If you prefer not to push yourself too hard, approximately 150 minutes a week (that is about 20 minutes a day) of moderate aerobic activity, will usually be enough to keep you healthy and provide you with the benefits I mentioned before. This type of exercise should leave you slightly breathless, but you should still be able to speak effortlessly.

Moderate activity includes exercises such as brisk walking, cycling or dancing. And If you want your exercise to be useful in other ways, mowing the lawn or cleaning the house would count too. Swimming is also a valuable activity, especially if you are suffering from any type of joint pain, as the water buoys you up while you are active.

Vigorous-Intensity Activity

If you prefer to pack your activity into a shorter time, you will only need 75 minutes a week of vigorous-intensity activity for the same effect as 150 minutes at a moderate level. This type of physical activity will make you very breathless and prevent you from having a conversation. That is approximately ten minutes a day. Can you commit ten minutes of your time every day for the sake of having good health?

This type of activity can include running, speed cycling or hill cycling, as well as walking up a staircase. Sports that involve running, such as football, rugby or hockey, will count, as will gymnastics, martial arts or aerobics.

High-Intensity Interval Training (HIIT)

HIIT is an extra vigorous activity, alternating short bursts of intense anaerobic exercise with periods of moderate activity, such as walking (e.g. 30 seconds of intense exercise and 15 seconds of moderate exercise). It is important not to overdo HIIT. Sessions should certainly not be longer than 30 minutes at a time unless you are already extremely fit.

HIIT activities can include lifting heavy weights or circuit training. It can also involve interval running or sprinting up hills or stairs.

Muscle Strengthening Exercise

Muscle strengthening is not only for bodybuilders. It is a good idea to include it in any exercise regime. You can lift heavy weights, work with resistance bands or do press-ups or sit-ups, for instance, either in the gym or at home.

There are other ways of strengthening your muscles, such as doing yoga, tai-chi or pilates. Alternatively, you can simply take advantage of everyday opportunities, including digging your garden, carrying heavy shopping or even carrying tired kids. It all counts.

Doing any of these types of exercise on a regular basis can help you improve your health and maintain your fitness level.

Combining exercise with a healthy diet is the best way to achieve a healthy and fit body.

How to Get Fit in 20 Minutes or Less?

Daily exercise of 20 minutes does not sound like a lot, does it? In essence, it is not, and those 20 minutes can change your life.

Just 20 minutes of your day dedicated to exercise could lead to a healthier you. What this means is: weight loss, increased energy levels, a toned and lean body, a better mood, improved heart health and all manner of other benefits, which I am sure will be welcome in your life.

You can have all of these benefits in just 20 minutes.

How Do You Do It?

It is about having the right blend of exercise for you.

In this book, I have shared 25 exercises. They work with every part of your body, from your shoulders to your toes. You do not need to complete all of them every day. You can choose which exercises you want to do each day and you can select the most suitable time of the day to do them. I am sure just 20 minutes a day will be manageable to fit into your life, no matter how busy you are.

I want to warn you that if you have a particular injury or mobility problem, seek out advice from your doctor or physio and tweak specific moves, so they do not harm or hurt you. All exercises can be modified. So, that is great news if you want to dedicate yourself to exercise and become fitter. Some exercises will require you to lift your leg high. If you feel pain in any part of your body, you might choose to lift your leg only halfway until your condition improves and you are able to challenge your body.

Try to start your workout with a few minutes of warm-up. It is important not to miss this step. Otherwise, you might end up with a muscle strain causing you some pain. Your warm-up can include running or jogging on the spot or jumping up and down. If you are unable to do any of these, then marching on the spot is a good alternative. You need to get your heart rate up and a little sweat going. Once you are feeling warm and your breathing is just a little faster than usual, you are ready to start working on each part of your body gradually.

It Is All About Toning

In the following chapter, we are going to cover some upper and lower body exercises that will not only work out the major muscles groups in each area but will keep the cardio element going. These exercises will also increase your flexibility and balance while at the same time working out your core.

The next chapter is about strength training. If you have some hand weights or small dumbbells, these will come in very handy and help you to tone your body a little faster. If you do not have these, a can of food will do the job just as well!

Once you finish your workout, spend the last few minutes cooling down with some stretches. You need to cool down your body just as much as you need to warm it up.

That is all it takes. Only 20 minutes of your day and over time you will start seriously noticing the difference. You will feel better, look fitter, and you will be healthier and stronger for it.

The good news is you do not need expensive gym membership for this either, all you need is a little bit of floor space in the comfort of your own home!

Chapter 2: Get Fit In the Comfort of Your Home

"People find it hard to fit exercise into their working-day life. Nine to five jobs take up most of your day, so it is always difficult. But a little can go a long way. It can be 10 or 15 minutes of exercise that can be of real benefit."

Laura Trott

In this chapter, I will share with you five types of exercise that you can do in your own home. You will not need any type of gym equipment to do them properly and they can be easily performed by beginners and more advanced athletes. Some exercises will require you to use a chair or a bench or two cans of food instead of a set of dumbbells. You will not need to spend any money and you will not even need to leave your home. All you will need is the commitment to improve yourself.

148

There are 25 exercises organised into five groups, with five different exercises in each group. These five groups include warm-up exercises, upper body exercises, lower body exercises, strength training and stretching. All of them play important roles and work with different parts of your body.

This plan is flexible, and it does not require you to spend any money, it is not time-consuming, and it shows you how to get great results with exercising in less than 20 minutes a day.

There are some simple rules to follow:

- Do not stick to doing only one type of exercise every day. Each activity provides you with different kinds of benefits. So, make sure that over time, you include them all in your workout. Doing this can also help you reduce boredom and the risk of injury.
- You can choose to do two or three exercises from each exercise group one day and then different exercises the following day.
- You may decide to focus only on stretching exercises one or two days a week, to give your body a rest.
- Feel free to approach your new exercise regime whichever way suits you. You can choose to do your 20 minutes of exercising in the morning, or during your lunch break, or in the evening after work. You may decide to split this time into two parts and exercise for ten minutes in the morning and another ten minutes in the evening. The most important thing is to stay consistent. Do it regularly and do not give up.

The purpose of exercise is to make you feel good, and that is what you will achieve after you consistently repeat what I am teaching you. You will feel better, mentally and physically. You will also start to feel better about yourself. You will experience this only if you include exercise in your daily routine. Very soon you will notice the difference in the way you look and most importantly, the way you feel. Spending 20 minutes a day on self-care is not too long. It is only a small fraction of a day. Think about all the benefits that you can achieve within such short period of ime. I am sure that some days you may not feel like exercising, but I am encouraging you to do it anyway. Your body will thank you for it.

Warm-Up Exercises

Warm-up exercises prepare the body for exercise. They help increase the blood flow to your muscles and loosen your joints. They can prevent injuries, boost your metabolism and increase muscle temperature. They also increase your energy productions. Warm-up exercises are great for reducing muscle pain.

Running/Marching on the Spot

Warming up is vital, and one of the easiest ways to do this is to try running on the spot or marching. Anyone can do this. You can vary the intensity according to your general health and any injuries you may have that you are trying to protect.

Benefits:

- Easy to do for anyone

- Warms up the body for cardiovascular exercise and strength training

- Works out all the major muscle groups

How to do it:

- Stand on the spot with your body upright and your shoulders back

- Start jogging or marching on the spot

- Lift your knees up as high as your hips

- Start to pump your arms up and down, moving them in the same rhythm as your feet

- Continue for 3 minutes

Knee Bends

You must protect your knees during any exercise. You can do this by bending your knees slightly whenever you do a workout on your lower body. However, warming up the muscles surrounding your knees is vital.

Benefits:

- Helps to warm up the muscles surrounding the knees

- Warms up the body for lower body exercise

- Raising your arms also warms up the upper body

- Easy to do

How to do it:

- Stand up straight with your legs shoulder width apart and elbows bent

- Gently bend your knees, pushing your buttocks slightly back

- Do not bend your knees too much (see the picture)

- Slowly return to your standing position

- Repeat two sets 8-10 times

Jumping Jack

Jumping jack is a popular aerobic exercise and great for a total-body workout. It is an excellent fat burning exercise. I suggest you try to incorporate it into your morning routine. Doing so will help you get in shape and soon you will notice the difference to your fitness level.

Benefits:

- Raises your heart rate and helps with weight loss

- Improves your mobility and circulation

- Works your heart, lungs and muscle

- Firms your glutes and calves

- Maintains your fitness level and helps you get in shape

- Helps you work on your biceps and triceps when slightly bending your arms

How to do it:

- Stand up straight with your legs together and arms at your sides

- Gently bend your knees and jump

- As you jump, spread your legs and stretch your arms as you can see in the picture

- Repeat this process for two minutes, try to do as many jumping jack's as you can during this time

- You can also repeat this jumping jack exercise several times a day for two minutes each time

Mountain Climber

This total-body workout is a great exercise for engaging your joints and muscles. It focuses on all of the body, from your neck down. Therefore, it works on many muscles at the same time. For this reason, it is a great warm-up exercise that can help you with your fitness level and overall health.

Benefits:

- Helps speed up your heart rate and supports the burning of calories and fat

- Helps with weight loss

- Helps build cardio endurance and strengthens the core

- Targets the abdominal muscles and builds triceps and shoulder muscles

- Works on quads and helps tone the glutes and hamstrings

How to do it:

- Lay down on your stomach, lift your body off the ground and keep your hips down

- Bring one knee to your chest, then pull it out

- Switch legs, and bring your other knee to your chest as much as you can, while you pull the other leg out

- Start slowly and then increase the speed, until you run against the floor

- Do a set of 10-15 in a row if you are a beginner and 25-30 if you are more advanced

Cross Body Toe Touches

This is an excellent exercise for people of any age and any fitness level. It involves many muscles, but it mainly focuses on the oblique muscle.

Benefits:

- Involves many muscles at the same time

- Works many muscles: obliques, shoulders, lower back, glutes and hamstring

- Great for your abdominal muscles and improving the strength of your core

- Stretches your back and hamstring

How to do it:

- Stand up straight with your legs shoulder-width apart

- Raise your arms to the sides as shown in the picture

- Bend down and touch your left toe with your right hand

- Keep rotating your body to the left and then to the right, reaching your toe with the opposite hand

- If you are not able to touch your toes, you can bend your knees slightly. The goal of this exercise is to rotate your body as fast as you can and squeeze your oblique muscle as hard as you can

- Do this exercise as fast as you can for one to two minutes

Upper Body Exercises

There are many health benefits of having a strong upper body. It can help heart health and improve your posture. The strong upper body plays a significant role in improving your flexibility and mobility as well as helping you to do a range of movements.

Shoulder Exercise – Power Partials

For this high-intensity exercise, you may want to get a set of dumbbells. These are easily available. If you do not have dumbbells, do not worry, you can use tins of food, which I am sure you can find them in your kitchen cupboard. You simply need a small set of hand weights to work out your upper body and arms with ease.

Benefits:

- Gives you a cardiovascular workout and helps with balance

- Engages the core muscles to add strength

- Focuses on the pectorals, the triceps and biceps

How to do it:

- Stand up straight with your feet shoulder-width apart and take your dumbbells/tins of food in your hands

- When you are ready, raise your arms out to the sides, level with your shoulders

- Hold the position for a few seconds and then lower your arms to your hips

- Repeat this process 12-15 times

- When you are ready to take this exercise to the next level and make it harder, instead of bringing your arms down to your hips, raise your arms straight above your head, hold them there for a few seconds and return to the shoulder height

- Repeat 15-20 times

Plank Leg Lifts

If you want an exercise which targets several major muscles all at one time, the plank leg lifts are a great choice. This is a great full-body exercise, but I decided to include it in this section as it is an excellent exercise for strengthening and toning your arms. While performing this exercise, focus on looking forward, rather than down, as it will help you straighten your body and keep your spine as flat as possible.

Benefits:

- Ideal for increasing your core strength

- Tones your whole body, especially your legs and arms

- Works out the abdominal muscles

- Stretches the hamstrings and glutes

- Improves your posture

- Burns fat

- Boosts your metabolism

How to do it:

- Lay down on your stomach, bend your hands under your shoulders and lift your body

- Rest your weight on your hands and the tips of your toes and engage your glutes and the core muscles when doing this

- Lift your right leg to a 45-degree angle and hold for 10 seconds

- Repeat ten times with each leg

Push-Ups

Everyone knows how to do a push-up, but are you sure you are doing them correctly? Push-ups help to boost your upper body strength and again, you simply need a little spare space on the floor to do them.

Benefits:

- Works out several major muscle groups, including the triceps, deltoids and pectorals

- Targets your core muscles and helps to build muscle mass over time

- Improves cardiovascular health

- Ideal for overall health and well-being

How to do it:

- Lay down on your stomach and place your hands under your shoulders

- Push upwards into a plank and then extend your arms, so your upper body is higher than your lower body

- Bend your elbows and lower your chest towards the floor

- Push up through your hands to move upwards, straightening out your arms

- Repeat three sets of 10 push-ups

- To make this exercise a little easier, keep your knees on the floor and lower your chest to the mat instead

Chair Push-Ups

If you find regular push-ups difficult, these chair push-ups may help you to tone the major arm muscles and your chest, while making the whole experience so much easier. You will need a chair or a stool to be placed against the wall, or in a position which means it is not going to slip when you put pressure on it. Also, wear shoes as they will give you a better grip.

Benefits:

- Targets shoulders and tones the arm muscles

- Great workout for your chest

- A good cardiovascular workout

- Increases strength and endurance

- Helps to improve your balance

How to do it:

- Place your stool or chair in a place where it is not going to slip and put your hands flat on it; keep your legs extended behind you and your body in a straight line

- Raise yourself on to your tiptoes and steady yourself, engaging your core muscles

- Ensure your palms are directly underneath your shoulders, then bend your elbows a little and lower your chest down towards the chair or stool

- Push up through your palms to raise and straighten your arms

- Repeat three sets of 10 push-ups

Triceps Dips with a Bench/Chair

A great bodyweight exercise that helps with building the strength of your arms and shoulders. You can do this workout anywhere; in the park, the kitchen or even in the office. All you need is a bench, a chair or steps.

Benefits:

- Works with your chest

- Strengthen the muscles in your triceps, chest and shoulders

- Tones your upper body

How to do it:

- Sit on the edge of the chair/bench and extend your legs hip-width apart, with heels touching the ground

- Look straight ahead with your chin up

- Slide slightly forward and lower yourself down as much as you can or until your elbows are 45-90 degrees

- Slowly push yourself to the starting position and repeat

- Do three sets of 10-15 push-ups and increase it to three sets of 20-30 times over four weeks

- If you find this exercise too hard, then bend your knees and move your feet closer to your body, until you increase your strength and you are able to do it with your legs extended

Lower Body Exercises

Building the strength of your lower body can hugely improve your balance, boost metabolism and reduce pain in your lower back. There are a number of exercises that you can do for your lower back. In this book, I have included the five most common exercises that support your lower body.

Squats

Squats help to tone and strengthen your lower body. If you want to tone your buttocks and thighs, then a series of squats is the ideal option for you.

Benefits:

- Tones the buttocks and thighs

- Works out the entire lower body

- Targets the core muscles

- A great cardiovascular workout

- Helps to improve balance

How to do it:

- Stand up straight with your feet in line with your hips

- Keep arms by your side

- Keep your back straight and your chest upwards

- Slowly bend your knees and push your hips backwards

- Your thighs should now be parallel to the floor

- Hold for a second and then push up through your heels to return to your original position

- Do three sets of 12 squats

Lunges

Lunges are a well-known exercise that is ideal for boosting the strength of major leg muscles, but they are also an excellent workout for the heart and cardiovascular system too. The good news is that you only need a little room in your living room to do them!

Benefits:

- Works out the major leg muscles, including the hamstrings and quads

- Helps to strengthen and tone the gluteal muscles

- Gives a great cardiovascular workout

- Improves balance

How to do it:

- Stand up straight with your arms relaxed by your sides or have them in front of you like shown in the picture

- Stride forwards with your right foot

- Bend both knees at a 90-degree angle

- Push your power back through your right foot to return to your original standing position

- Repeat ten times on your right leg and another ten times on your left leg

Side Lunges

Side lunges are a great way to work out your abductor muscles. The same as a regular lunge but working to the side instead, just make sure that you have plenty of space around you when you attempt this exercise.

Benefits:

- Works the abductor muscles

- A great cardiovascular workout

- Will help to increase your balance and flexibility

- Works out your core muscles at the same time

How to do it:

- Stand up straight and take a big step to your right side

- Slow drop down into a lunge so that your right leg is bent at a 90-degree angle

- Keep your left leg straight

- Push through your heel to return to your original position

- Repeat on your right leg ten times

- Repeat the exercise ten times with your left leg

Pistol Squats

If you want to turn up the heat and give yourself the best toning exercise, pistol squats are the way to go. It is a tough exercise, so you may need to take it slowly at first.

Benefits:

- A great cardiovascular exercise

- Focuses on the quads, hamstrings and the gluteal muscles

- Will add strength to your lower body quickly

- Increases your flexibility and balance

How to do it:

- Stand up straight, with your arms at your sides or in front of you like shown in the picture

- Place your weight on one leg and drop down into a squat, as low as you can go without losing your balance

- As you do, point the other leg out straight in front of you

- Repeat ten times on the same leg

- Switch to the other leg and repeat ten times

Side-Lying Leg Lift

The side-lying leg lift focuses on the lower body and works with many groups of muscles. If you find it too challenging to perform this exercise, you can do the leg lift standing up, instead of lying down. Once you improve your strength, then you can do the leg lift lying down.

Benefits:

- Focuses on many muscles of your lower body

- Works on glutes, hips, hamstrings, calves, obliques and tights

- Tones your legs, core and butt

- Works with the hip muscles

How to do it:

- Lie down on your side and place one arm under your head and rest the other arm on your hip

- Your top leg should be lying on top of your other leg

- Raise your top leg as high as you can

- Keep your spine straight while doing this exercise

- Lower your top leg down and repeat

- When finished, lie on the other side of the body and repeat this exercise with your other leg

- Start with three sets of 10-15 leg lifts for each leg, until you feel comfortable doing between 20-25 or more lifts with each leg

Strength Training Exercises

Strength training can help your health in many ways. It can make your body stronger, leaner and fitter. It is excellent for your bone health and for improving muscle mass. It offers excellent support to manage chronic diseases such as diabetes, arthritis and cardiovascular disease. It is not uncommon to notice an improvement in energy levels and mood after engaging in a strength training exercise, due to the increased level of endorphins which are released by doing the workout. For weight loss, it is recommended to do regular strength training. Numbers of studies show that strength training can speed up your metabolism, which is responsible for helping manage your weight.

Side Plank

The side plank helps to strengthen your core and abdominal muscles, therefore helping you with your balance and general health and well-being. The side plank is the ideal exercise to try. You might not be able to hold it for too long at first, but the more you practice, the longer you will be able to do it. The side plank will not only add strength to your muscles, but you will also increase your balance and flexibility at the same time.

Benefits:

- Works out your core muscles and strengthens all abdominal muscles, including obliques

- Works out your back muscles at the same time

- Great for toning the arms and the inner thighs

- Increases your balance

- Excellent for building your strength in general

How to do it:

- Lay down on one side, put your elbow underneath your shoulder, and place your left foot on top of your right foot

- Keep your feet together and push up your arms and your hips off the floor until you are balancing on your arm and tiptoes

- Hold for a while and relax, before repeating

- If you want to add an extra challenge, try it with a straight arm and raise your opposite arm towards the ceiling, as shown in the picture

- Slowly build up the length of time you can hold the plank

V Sit

You might also hear this called the "boat pose." If you want to give your core muscles the best workout possible, the V sit is a great option. You can initially start holding the V sit for around ten seconds. Then slowly work up to longer increments.

Benefits:

- Works out your core muscles very well

- Focuses on the lower abdominals and the lower back

- Great for working out the hip flexors

- Improves your balance and core strengthen overall

- An excellent cardiovascular workout at the same time

How to do it:

- Lay down on either the ground or a mat

- At the same time, slowly lift your legs (keeping them together) and your upper body, so you form a V shape

- Lift your arms pointing towards your raised legs, to give extra support

- If you want to make it a little easier, bend your legs but raise your feet off the floor

- Hold for ten seconds initially

- Build up to 20 and 30-second increments

Wall Dips

You need to be near a wall for this exercise. You can build up the amount of time you hold the pose for, depending upon how strong you are to begin with. This exercise also gives you a little cardio workout too.

Benefits:

- Works the core muscles and adds strength

- Helps with flexibility and balance

- Gives a cardio element to your workout

- Targets the lower body, including the gluteals, calves, hamstrings and the inner thighs

How to do it:

- Stand up straight with your back against the wall

- Slowly slide your upper back down the wall and bend your legs, so you are in a sitting position

- You should be holding all your weight on your legs

- Hold it for as long as you can, start at ten seconds and build up to longer durations, breath steadily as you go, and repeat a few times

- If you want to make the exercise a little more difficult, get a ball and hold it between your knees

Step up Onto a Chair

This exercise will support you to improve your balance and offer you many health benefits. It is also good for strengthening different muscles in your body. This exercise requires you to have a sturdy chair or a bench.

Benefits:

- Exercises the whole body

- Targets the hamstring, quadriceps and glutes

- Tones your legs and buttocks

- Strengthens and tones the entire body

- Helps you to lose weight

- Improves your balance

How to do it:

- Step in front of the chair/bench

- Place the right foot on the chair/bench and then step on it

- Put both of your feet on the floor one by one

- Then repeat with your left foot first

- Repeat as many as you can in 30 seconds

Bird-Dog Exercise

This simple core exercise is excellent for your spine and can support your posture and help reduce lower back pain.

Benefits:

- Strengthen the core and hips

- Works on your back muscle

- Improves your stability

How to do it:

- Get on the floor on your knees

- Keep your spine straight

- Raise your left arm and left leg, keep your shoulders and hips parallel to the floor

- Stay in this position for approximately five seconds and then go back to the starting position

- Then raise your right arm and left leg

- Do two to three sets of 10 times on each side

Stretching

You can do stretching before or after athletic activity or you can do it on its own. There are a number of benefits that you can gain from doing stretching and it is advisable to include it in your daily routine. Stretching is excellent for keeping muscles healthy and strong. Other benefits include improved flexibility, better posture and higher performance in physical activities. It can also help with back pain and relieve stress levels. Stretching helps your body as well as your mind.

Hamstring Stretches

The hamstring muscles are one of the most commonly injured muscles in the body, so it is not only essential to warm them up before exercising, but also to give them a good stretch afterwards. This particular exercise is ideal for that.

Benefits:

- Works out and stretches the hamstrings

- Increases balance

- A relaxing exercise to finish off your workout

How to do it:

- Lay down on your back with your arms by your sides and both legs fully stretched out

- Start with the right leg first; hold the back of your right knee with both hands and pull it toward your chest

- Slowly straighten the knee until it feels as it is stretching

- Keep your back straight throughout

- Hold the stretch for 10-30 seconds

- Repeat with your left leg

Seated Toe Stretches

This is a great stretching exercise that helps with better flexibility. Having better flexibility can improve your mobility and posture. Flexible muscles can decrease the risks of some injuries.

Benefits:

- Improves your physical performance

- Helps with flexibility

- Supports your mobility

How to do it:

- Sit on the floor with your legs straight

- Lift your toes and try to touch them with your hands as shown in the picture

- When you reach your toes, hold for five seconds, and relax

- Repeat 10-15 times

Quad Stretches

If you want to stretch out your quads and increase your balance at the same time, squad stretches are perfect. This can be done before exercise or afterwards, as part of your warm-down.

Benefits:

- Stretches out the quads

- Increases your balance

- Improves flexibility

How to do it:

- Stand up straight, with loose shoulders

- Bring your right leg up, bending backwards until it touches your bottom

- Keep your straight leg slightly bent at the knee

- Take hold of your leg with your right arm

- When you are ready and if you want to, push your hips slightly forwards

- Hold the stretch for 30 seconds, then repeat with your left leg

- If you need a little help with balancing, you can hold onto the wall or a chair with your opposite arm

Hip Flexor Stretching

Hip flexor stretching is ideal for you if you are spending long hours sitting down. An inactive lifestyle can cause your hip flexors to become tight and this can cause problems of your lower back.

Benefits:

- Can prevent back pain

- Can prevent hip pain

How to do it:

- Get down on your knee

- Place your feet as shown in the picture; one foot is underneath your body, while the other foot is behind you

- Lean forwards while you are squeezing your buttocks

- Hold it for approximately one minute

- Repeat with your other leg

- If you spend long hours every day sitting down, you can do this exercise 2-3 times a day, this will help to prevent pain developing in your hips and the lower back

Bent-Arm Shoulder Stretch

An inactive lifestyle, stress and some physical activities, can cause stress to your body. Most of us tend to hold the most tension in our shoulders and tight shoulders can cause us to experience pain in our neck, back and upper body. This shoulder stretching exercise can prevent stiffness and help you become more flexible.

Benefits:

- Stretches several muscles on the side of your upper body

- Stretches your triceps

- Stretches your shoulders

How to do it:

- Stand up or sit down and keep your body straight

- Raise your left arm, bend it to 90 degrees and place it behind your neck

- Use your right arm to gently push the elbow of your left arm behind your back

- Hold the stretch in this position for a minimum of 30 seconds

- Relax and repeat this process with your other arm

Chapter 3: Diet

"A healthy outside starts from the inside."

Rober Urich

Benefits of Healthy Eating

Exercise is vital for good health and weight loss, but it is unlikely to be much of a bonus if you are eating unhealthily.

To lose weight, many people start exercising by going to the gym, running or engaging in another type of physical activity. However, not many people understand why they are still not losing weight, even though they exercise regularly. An inability to lose weight could be down to a bad diet, an inactive lifestyle, hormonal imbalance, too much stress or another factor. If you are struggling to lose weight, I cannot confirm the reason for it, but one thing I can confirm is that you cannot out-train a bad diet. To burn off two slices of pizza, you will need to run for at least half an hour. The problem is that not many people settle for only two slices of pizza. They also may have garlic bread, a glass of wine and maybe a dessert. In addition to other foods and drinks consumed throughout the day this can lead to consuming too many calories in one day.

Healthy eating and exercising should never be only about weight loss. Health must always be your primary focus. I understand that junk food might taste good and that healthy eating could be confusing, hard and even inconvenient for some people (not to mention boring), but those are just unconscious excuses. Once you start eating healthy food, you will not want to go back to your old diet. I would also like to say that in my opinion, healthy food tastes delicious, you just need to know how to cook it.

Let's look at the benefits of healthy eating. They tend to range from physical to mental benefits. Here are the main ones.

Weight Loss and Disease Prevention

Losing weight is the most common motivation to go on a healthy diet. It can be vital for your psychological well-being since body image has a powerful effect on how happy we are. However, the benefits do not stop there.

Being overweight or obese can increase your risk of many serious diseases and reaching your optimal weight can significantly reduce this risk. Heart disease and strokes, for example, are associated with unhealthy eating and obesity.

Recent research in Canada has suggested that a healthy weight-loss diet can prevent these diseases in 80% of cases.

Similarly, losing weight through healthy eating can help with the management of type 2 diabetes and there is evidence that both a healthy weight and a healthy diet can reduce the risk of developing some types of cancer.

Benefits to the Body's Health

Many aspects of your body need to function at an optimal level for you to be and feel healthy and both these aspects are often significantly improved by healthy eating.

The food you eat is what the body uses to continue building itself, including your bones and teeth. If you ensure your diet includes the various minerals required for this, you are reducing the risk of developing osteoporosis and osteoarthritis in later life.

Similarly, a healthy gut is vital for both health and well-being. A diet rich in prebiotics and probiotics can strengthen the friendly bacteria in your gut, which not only boosts your metabolism, but also fights harmful bacteria and can even reduce the risk of bowel cancer.

Benefits to Mental Health

As mentioned previously, achieving your target weight can have a powerful psychological effect, leaving you feeling much happier and more positive. However, healthy eating can also have more direct benefits on your mood, since some unhealthy foods can contribute to depression and fatigue.

Eating healthy has also been linked with improving brain function. In the short term, this can improve memory, but in the long run, there are suggestions it could also reduce the risk of cognitive decline and dementia as you get older.

If all this is not enough, a healthy diet can also improve your sleep pattern. So, this benefits both your physical and mental health, as well as helping you enjoy a better lifestyle.

What Is a Healthy Diet?

We have established how crucial it is for both your physical and mental well-being, to eat healthily. But what exactly is a healthy diet?

According to the NHS, a healthy diet means "Eating a wide variety of foods in the right proportions and consuming the right amount of food and drink to achieve and maintain a healthy body weight." While fad diets are not healthy, they area type of diet that focus on limiting food choices and calorie restriction.

What Varieties of Food Should You Be Eating?

There are five primary food groups and all of them are a part of a healthy diet. Some of the foods come from meat or dairy and if you are either a vegetarian or vegan, there are alternatives available.

- Protein-rich foods, including meat, fish, eggs, beans and pulses, are essential for the body to grow and repair, as well as providing iron, zinc and B vitamins. In the case of meat, poultry is ideal, though lean cuts of other meats are acceptable, I suggest you avoid processed meat as much as possible.
- It is essential to eat at least five portions of fruit and vegetables a day, which can be fresh, dried, tinned or frozen, to provide a range of vitamins and minerals. Vegetables should make up a substantial part of each meal. There is evidence this can lead to a lower risk of strokes and heart disease.
- Starchy foods, which contain fibre, vitamins and minerals, should make up a third of your diet. More natural forms are healthier like brown rice, whole-wheat pasta, wholemeal bread and potatoes with their skins on.
- Milk, cheese and yoghurt are good sources of protein and calcium, which strengthen your bones. If your diet is dairy-free, alternatives such as soy-based milk and plant-based cheese can give similar benefits.
- Some fat is essential, but make sure you use it in small quantities. Some oils, such as olive oil, are excellent sources of unsaturated fat, which supply the body with fatty acids to absorb vitamins. Saturated fat is not the best option. It usually comes from animal products such as fatty pieces of beef or pork. I want to mention here that coconut oil also contains saturated fat, but

as it is a plant, it can provide you with many health benefits. Trans fat can be found in foods such as cakes and biscuits and is the type of fat that you need to steer away from.

Also, it is vital to drink plenty of fluids during the day, the majority of which should be water. Restrict caffeinated and alcoholic drinks to a minimum. Drinking too much alcohol can weaken your immune system and increase the risk of certain diseases such as a stroke, high blood pressure and a heart attack. There are also many side effects of consuming large amounts of caffeinated drinks, which include insomnia, caffeine addiction and high blood pressure.

Eat Sensibly

It is essential to include all these food groups in your daily diet. Some of the foods, such as starch and fat, have traditionally been regarded as causing weight gain. In fact, this is more to do with specific sources, such as white bread and saturated or trans fats. Swapping these for a healthier option in the same group will help towards maintaining your ideal weight.

In general, the fresher and less prepared your ingredients are, the better for you. Although, as noted, frozen or tinned vegetables are often a good substitute. One advantage of preparing meals from scratch is that you always know what is going in them.

This does not mean you cannot eat fast food meal or a cake ever again, but these foods should be left for specific occasions and used as special treats. Then the following day you can return to your healthy diet again.

What Is the Difference Between a Healthy Diet and a Weight Loss Diet?

We hear a lot about fad diets, but these are the types of so-called diets you need to avoid at all costs. The problem is that many dieters follow this type of diet regularly with the hope that it will help them lose weight.

Some of these diets are extremely dangerous as they do not provide the body with essential nutrients needed for healthy functioning. They tend to focus too much on weight loss and do not pay much attention to health.

To lose weight fast, many people become obsessed with counting calories and this often leads to starvation. So, the weight-loss diet actually turns into a hunger diet.

Generally, weight-loss diets are very restrictive. In addition to removing a fair amount of food you consume daily, dieters also stop eating all the foods they love the most. After doing this for a few days or weeks, dieting becomes a chore that is not sustainable and is very hard to follow. The combination of starvation and deprivation never brings positive results.

It is important to remember there is no such thing as quick weight loss. If you want to lose weight permanently, you need to do it steadily. That means focusing on around 1-2 lb or 1 kg of steady loss every week. You should do this by eating healthy foods, varying your diet and exercising regularly.

A healthy diet is as we know a lifestyle choice. It means focusing on clean, natural and fresh foods, lean meats, avoiding sugary foods and high-fat options and steering clear of processed foods. That does not mean you cannot have the odd treat, of course you can, but it should all be in moderation. When you add exercise into that type of lifestyle, you will lose weight, albeit slowly. The plus point of this is that you are more likely to keep the weight off and you will feel far better in yourself too.

There tends to be a big difference between a healthy diet and a weight-loss diet, but it should not be that way. The intention of both diets should be to provide you with healthy nutrients that nourish your body. The issue is that a weight-loss diet often does not do this.

A healthy diet is focusing on the quality of food you consume, while the weight-loss diet is more focused on restricting and minimising the quantity of foods you eat, sometimes to an unhealthy level. When eating healthy, you end up being healthy as well as slim. Therefore, a healthy diet with exercise is always the best route forwards, there is no question about that, whether your goal is to lose weight or to be healthy.

How to Prepare Healthy Meals in Minutes?

In a world that is becoming increasingly defined by complexity and more activity than you can manage to fit into your 24-hour day, it is becoming increasingly difficult to cook a decent meal. We face mounting deadlines and delivery periods that sometimes loom over our heads like a dark cloud.

Some days, you might not even get to eat at all and on other days you may rely on processed foods or start binging on everything from packaged snacks to beverages. While studies continue to point you to the dangers of depending on processed and packaged foods, you see it, but there is nothing much you can do, you think. You want to live healthier, but the speed and mounting pressure that defines your week and life do not allow you to. You have even made plans and resolutions, but the timeline for making that transition from your junk food lifestyle to a more healthier living just keeps moving further away.

How to Make a Start

I understand your dilemma, and I can see your difficulties in this regard. However, making a healthy and nutritious meal is not as time-consuming as you have got yourself conditioned to believe. With the right meal ideas and different meal combinations to follow, you will very quickly get yourself on a healthy diet while also achieving your deadlines.

Many people believe that eating healthy is expensive, time-consuming or hard to learn, not realising that their lack of knowledge influences these conclusions. If you are one of these people who hold such beliefs, well, then it is great that you are reading this book because you will soon learn that you can make healthy and nutritious meals in minutes. You will find out from the meal ideas I am sharing with you in this book, that living a healthy life lies within your reach and you only need to be pointed in the right direction. The meal ideas in this book are so simple and easy to make. You do not need to be a chef or a great cook to be able to prepare healthy meals and eat healthy. You just need to follow these meal ideas I am sharing with you and combine them with the exercises I have shared with you in the previous chapter.

Eating Healthy is Not So Hard

You see, nature has provided us with lots of fruits and vegetables. There are over 1000 edible plants that nourish our bodies. There are also various animal proteins and food supplements that can make us healthy and deliver all the nutrients that our bodies need. So, whether you are vegan, vegetarian or love those chicken wings, you can find a space for your appetite. Living healthily does not require you to break the bank or exceed your budget as the meal combinations and suggestions I will be giving you are both pocket friendly and readily available; talk about having your cake and eating it.

In the next chapter you will find lots of simple meal ideas. They are highly nutritious and focused to get you powering through your schedule while living a healthy life. From breakfast to lunch to dinner and everything in-between, you can combine your need for speed with a convenient meal plan that put you on a healthy diet and a low budget.

A recipe book *Get Slim and Healthy in 20 Minutes or Less* is yours. It is your free bonus and a great addition to the book you are holding in your hands right now. Go to www.bit.ly/bundle-fit-and-healthy and download your free copy. You will discover lots of healthy and delicious recipes, designed to support you on your journey towards permanent weight loss and good health.

Chapter 4: Simple and Healthy Meal and Drink Ideas

"Good food is very often, even most often, simple food."

Anthony Bourdain

Eating and drinking in a healthy way does not have to be too hard or too confusing. You simply need a few ideas to get you on the right track.

Here are 9 healthy eating tips to get you started and lead you to your success, so you can reach your health and weight loss goals quickly.

Healthy Eating Tips

Start the day with breakfast.
Eat a variety of fruits and vegetables.
Eat lean protein and healthy fats, and try to include them with each meal, if possible.
Consume organic foods whenever possible.
Consume small portion sizes.
Eat frequent meals.
Drink plenty of water.
Do not eat late at night.
Enjoy what you eat!

Simple and Healthy Breakfast Ideas

I am sure you have heard of a famous quote by Adelle Davis, an American author and nutritionist, known for her work in the early to mid-20th century, "Eat breakfast like a king, lunch like a prince and dinner like a pauper."

Since your younger days to much of your adult life, the cliché "breakfast is the most important meal of the day" has been communicated in many different ways. This message remains as important today, as it is correct. As true as it is, however, the most flouted meal of the day is breakfast, and the reason is simple. The mad dash to get out of the door and the daily hustle and bustle of life has effectively made it impossible for many people to have their breakfast, or to put it mildly, a healthy breakfast.

I suggest you try to make some time in the morning to fill your body with the necessary nutrients. Your body will thank you for it. Filling your body with the right fuel at the beginning of each day will help you to feel healthier and more energised. A healthy breakfast will prevent you from reaching for sugary snacks at around 11 a.m. or carbohydrate rich foods for lunch.

Below are some breakfast ideas that would fit into your ever-shrinking time, ensuring that you do not have to skip the most important meal of the day anymore.

Fruit smoothie – Simply place a selection of your favourite fruits into a blender and add a little Greek yoghurt for a healthy and delicious start to your morning. This will kickstart your five a day challenge early on.

Mashed avocado on wholemeal toast – Avocado is packed with vitamins and minerals and it provides your body with healthy fats.

Granola with fruit and yoghurt – Granola will keep you fuller for longer, so you will avoid those mid-morning munchies. Add some berries and a little bit of yoghurt for a delicious and healthy start to the day. Most yoghurts are packed with sugar, therefore I recommend you read food labels. Greek yoghurt is high in protein, so it could be a great choice to have it with your first meal of the day.

Boiled eggs on wholemeal toast – Eggs are a great source of zinc, calcium, protein and all the major vitamin groups.

Wholemeal toast is a slow-release food, so it keeps you full throughout the morning.

Oatmeal with strawberries – If you are not a strawberry fan, you can add any other type of berry and you will be getting a good dose of vitamins and antioxidants, while the oatmeal will fill you up for longer which will prevent you from reaching for an unhealthy snack a couple of hours later.

Vegetable omelette – Use coconut oil, whisk up two eggs and add in your favourite vegetables, such as peppers, onions, tomatoes, mushrooms, etc. Coconut oil will provide your body with healthy fats, while the protein in the eggs will keep you full. You will also receive some antioxidant and vitamin benefits from the vegetables.

Overnight oats – You can have them with a fruit topping: a handful of fresh or frozen berries, grated apple, peach, plum or apricot, or you can have it with "good" fat topping: nut butter, pumpkin, sunflower seeds, etc.

Pancakes – You can find recipes for the variety of pancakes in the recipe book. Go to www.bit.ly/bundle-fit-and-healthy and download *Get slim and healthy in 20 minutes or less*. Depending on the type of pancakes you go for and the topping you choose (you will notice there is a nice variety there), you will receive many essential nutrients that will prepare your body for the day ahead.

Nut butter with a slice of rye bread – You will receive plenty of healthy nutrients with nut butter including protein, fibre, healthy fat as well as some vitamins and minerals. Due to the high nutrient content it is fine to consume nut butter, but only in moderate amount. Make sure you do not overdo it because of high amount of fat in nut butter. From rye bread, you will get plenty of fibre, iron and B vitamins. This can reduce inflammation and help with heart health and it can also support your weight loss.

Two slices of cold salmon, two scrambled eggs and one medium tomato – Salmon provides your body with Omega-3 fatty acids, protein, potassium and B vitamins. From eggs, you will get additional high-quality protein as well as many vitamins and minerals. Tomato is rich in antioxidants. Together, these foods will provide you with essential nutrients for your body to function at its best.

Slice of wholemeal toast with three tablespoons of low-sugar baked beans – Beans are a great source of plant-based protein that comes from seeds. They are high in minerals that provide you with energy and help boost your immune system.

Simple and Healthy Lunch Ideas

Lunch happens to be in the middle of the working day for most people. For this reason, many people do not pay much attention to the quality of the food they eat for lunch. They tend to grab whatever they can find in the local shop or a cafe. Here, I am sharing some ideas on what to eat for lunch and it includes a nice variety of food that you can easily prepare at home and take to work.

Lean chicken slices with lettuce, onion, tomatoes – Lean chicken is an excellent source of protein, which keeps you fuller for longer.

Tuna and jacket potato – Stick to a small potato and make sure you cook it in the oven for the best taste. Added tuna is rich in Omega-3, iron and magnesium.

Vegetable soup – Instead of buying tinned soup, I suggest you make it yourself to get the best vitamin content and add in as many vegetables as you enjoy. The more you include, the more vitamins and minerals you will receive and it is a hearty lunch that will keep you full until dinner.

Cauliflower pizza – Did you know that you can make a pizza base with cauliflower? This will make it far healthier from having a flour pizza base. Stick to a small amount of cheese and top with as many vegetables as you want.

Ratatouille – It is high in potassium, folate, fibre and vitamin C. It is very easy to take it to work and warm up in the microwave.

Lemon chicken pasta – Stick to wholemeal pasta and grill your chicken instead of frying it for a healthier twist. This meal traditionally has a creamy pasta sauce, but instead of the cream you can add coconut oil and add plenty of vegetables such as spinach, garlic and leaks. The lemon adds a tangy twist and a dose of vitamin C.

Large egg/tuna/grilled chicken salad – This is such a simple and healthy meal idea and it is so easy to prepare. Feel free to choose between the hard-boiled egg, tin of tuna or grilled chicken. Whatever you decide to have as your base, make sure you add a variety of vegetables. Here are some vegetables that you may want to include in your salad: red onion, spring onion, sweetcorn, cucumber, tomatoes, olives, grated carrot, pepper (red, yellow, orange or green), lettuce, spinach, radish, etc. Avoid using a creamy sauce such as mayonnaise or salad cream and instead, use a little bit of olive oil or vinegar. This meal will provide you with plenty of vitamins and minerals that you will gain from vegetables. In addition to this, you will get protein from the egg, tuna or chicken.

Large fruit salad with mix seeds – Some days you may not be too hungry and having a fruit salad for lunch might be sufficient. Prepare a bowl with chopped pieces of fruits such as an apple, nectarine, banana, grapes, watermelon, etc. and at the end, do not forget to add seeds such as pumpkin or sunflower seeds. Even though the fruits contain natural sugar, it is still a sugar and seeds can provide you with protein, healthy fats, fibre, alongside vitamins and minerals, which will help you keep your blood sugar balance stable.

Plain omelette with a large green salad – This simple meal will provide you with all the necessary nutrients: plenty of vitamins and minerals from the salad and protein from the eggs which will keep you full till snacktime or even dinnertime.

Soup – In my recipe book *Get slim and healthy in 20 minutes or less,* you will find a recipe for *Roasted red pepper and tomato soup.* It is easy and quick to prepare and is an excellent choice for a healthy lunch. You will receive all the healthy nutrients from the garlic, tomatoes, almonds, etc.

Wholemeal wrap with tomato, mozzarella and half an avocado – Avocado is a highly nutritious food. It may reduce your chances of developing heart disease and protect you from chronic illnesses, while mozzarella can support your bone health. A wholemeal wrap is a good source of magnesium, potassium and zinc. These vitamins are necessary for the healthy functioning of your body.

Simple and Healthy Dinner Ideas

If you have a long day at work and you are feeling tired by the time you get home, it is so easy to get a takeaway or grab a ready-made meal, or simply buy a sandwich and a bar of chocolate on the way home from work. This is not the best solution and you know it. Therefore, I am sharing with you some simple and healthy meal ideas. They are very easy and quick to prepare.

Jacket sweet potato with your favourite protein filling and green salad – Sweet potato is more nutritious and less fattening than a white jacket potato. It is high in antioxidants and I suggest you eat the potato skin as well, as it is a great source of fibre. Make sure you choose a small sweet potato and add any filling that is rich in protein. It can include tuna, cottage cheese or boiled egg. As a salad dressing, use a sprinkle of olive oil, vinegar or a spoon of squeezed lemon juice.

Baked salmon fillet with vegetables – Salmon is high in protein and rich in healthy fats. It is also high in vitamins and some minerals. Enjoy the fish with green beans, broccoli and three new potatoes.

Grilled fish with roast vegetables – Feel free to choose any white fish and have it with roasted vegetables such as courgettes, leek, peppers and a small portion of cooked brown rice or lentils.

Grilled lean chicken breast with salad – A piece of protein mixed with a few baby tomatoes, half an avocado, plenty of green salad and olive oil as a dressing.

Roasted vegetables – This is a delicious, healthy and easy meal to prepare. You can use the following vegetables: mushrooms, sliced red onions, tomatoes, courgettes, carrots, peppers, herbs, etc. Chop all the vegetables and drizzle with a little oil. When the vegetables are soft, serve them with couscous, which is a great and healthy alternative to pasta or rice. You will receive a high dose of vitamins and minerals to support your overall health. Tip: there is no need to peel courgettes or carrots. Skin of most vegetables is good for you. It will also save you time.

Vegetarian bolognese – Make your bolognese sauce with a small portion of mincemeat and plenty of vegetables. Serve with shaved courgettes instead of pasta. This meal is rich in a variety of nutrients and can help your heart health, digestion and support your weight loss.

Stuffed peppers and brown rice – The brighter the pepper, the higher the antioxidant level and when it is stuffed with brown rice and other vegetables, it is truly delicious. This meal is packed with a variety of vitamins and minerals and the brown rice will keep you fuller.

Garlic stuffed chicken – We all know that chicken is an easy meal and it is a great source of protein, but it can be boring on its own. So, you can cut it in half and stuff it with garlic and cook it in the oven. Garlic is high in iron, calcium, copper and potassium.

Grilled salmon, large salad and new potatoes – Salmon is high in Omega-3 fatty acids, magnesium, zinc and potassium, while also being very filling and delicious. Serve it with large salad and three new potatoes.

Balsamic chicken and asparagus – Simply marinade your chicken in delicious balsamic vinegar for a real kick and add in some asparagus. Not only do you get protein, but you are also getting all the major vitamin groups and fibre from the asparagus.

Eggplant lasagne – Just because you are trying to be healthy, it does not mean you have to give up your favourite food. Eggplant is a great meat substitute, in this case, make your own tomato sauce and use cheese sparingly for a delicious meal with calcium, vitamins C, K and B.

Simple and Healthy Snack Ideas

Dieters often try to avoid eating a snack but there is nothing wrong with snacking. They will keep you full and satisfied between main meals. The secret is to find what snacks are good for you. Here are some suggestions that will not only satisfy your hunger but will also provide you with healthy nutrients that your body needs. Once again, these are quick, simple and healthy.

Fresh fruit salad with yoghurt – As I already mentioned, you will find that yoghurts tend to be high in sugar. Learning how to read food labels is a must if you want to consume healthy foods. Choose soya yoghurt or Greek yoghurt, which are much healthier options. You can also sprinkle some seeds on top.

Mixed nuts – A handful of nuts can give you a high dose of healthy fats, protein and fibre. Nuts are also linked to a lower risk of heart disease and even prevent certain types of cancer.

Apple slices and peanut butter – Slice an apple and dip it (sparingly) into a little peanut butter. Peanut butter is linked to lowering blood cholesterol and apples are high in fibre. I already mentioned that a small amount of healthy fat is good for you, and you should avoid consuming too much fat.

Kale chips – Kale is super healthy and packed with antioxidants and fibre. You simply need to bake it until crispy.

Cherry tomatoes and mozzarella – From tomatoes, you are getting potassium, and vitamin C, as well as lycopene.

Mozzarella (in moderation) is high in protein and calcium. They are also delicious when combined together.

Hard-boiled eggs – We all know that eggs are very healthy, but they are also a great snack too. Rich in protein, vitamin B12 and K2, eggs will also keep you fuller until you reach lunch or dinnertime.

Olives – Olives can be enjoyed as part of a meal, but they are a great snack too. Olives are also high in healthy fats and antioxidants.

Two Oatcakes with hummus – Rich in protein, fibre and some minerals. They are a great choice to support your weight loss.
Six cubes of feta cheese and six olives – A great source of protein and healthy fats. It will decrease your hunger level between meals and keep your blood sugar levels stable.

Berries with a few nuts –Choose any type of berries and nuts. Berries are high in antioxidants, help with inflammation and are rich in fibre. Nuts are also a great source of fat, protein and fibre, and may also reduce the risk of having a heart attack or stroke.

Spicy nut mix – A great combination of nuts and spices that can provide you with plenty of health benefits. You can find this recipe in *Get slim and healthy in 20 minutes or less*. To download this 29-page recipe book, go to www.bit.ly/bundle-fit-and-healthy.

Simple and Healthy Drink Ideas

The majority of people are aware of what healthy food is, but they are less familiar with what a healthy drink is. So, they may eat healthily, but not drink healthy. Beverages such as Coke, Fanta and most energy drinks are packed with sugar and chemicals not recognisable by the human body and yet people still drink them, often in large amounts. Here are some examples of healthy drinks.

Water with a squeeze of fresh lime and lemon – Even diet versions of your favourite fizzy beverage are high in sweeteners and it is important to keep your body hydrated with as much water as you can. Add a squeeze of fresh lemon and lime to take away the blandness.

Lemon and ginger tea – A little fresh ginger and lemon mixed with hot water will give you a warm and healthy drink. You will get plenty of vitamin C, plus zinc, potassium, magnesium and iron.

Almond milk – Almond milk is a healthier and delicious alternative to regular milk, look for organic options to find the cleanest source possible.

Coconut milk – Coconut milk is a great source of calcium. It also contains magnesium, iron, vitamins C, E and B vitamins.

Turmeric tea – Turmeric is a superfood and contains more than 300 natural vitamins, minerals and other components which are vital for health. It is also delicious and gives you a herby and spicy tea to enjoy.

Fresh mint tea – Fresh mint leaves added to hot water provide a sweet flavour and give you plenty of health benefits, such as improving the symptoms of cold, helping with indigestion and they may also help with inflammation.

Green tea – Green tea is a great detoxing drink, but it is also packed with zinc, manganese and vitamins A to D.

Coconut water – Enjoy the tropical taste and receive vitamin C, B6, folate and plenty of potassium and magnesium.

Smoothie – Choose three different types of fruits, add some seeds and natural water. Mix everything in the blender and enjoy the nutrients that you can find in fruits and seeds.

Chapter 5: Live Healthy Every Day

"Try to think of working out and healthy eating as a lifestyle. Rather than go on a diet or try a crazy exercise routine, try making them something you do every day."

Allyson Felix

How to Establish a Healthy Daily Routine?

Routines are essential for us to function as human beings, allowing us to remember the numerous processes we have to go through in our lives. Routines are made of habits that we repeated a number of times and they have a strong impact on our lives. These sequences of repeated patterns, we tend to follow without much thought. We do them most of the time on autopilot.

However, due to this it is very easy to fall into routines that could have a harmful effect on our health and lives. Perhaps you have a habit of always buying a chocolate bar or bag of crisps on your way into work. Or maybe you habitually collapse in front of the TV when you get home.

This is the reason why establishing a healthy daily routine is vital to achieving a healthy lifestyle. You need to do it purposefully and for a more extended period, for it to be adopted as a part of your life. It is important to understand that working towards establishing your healthy daily routine could be challenging, but it might be necessary to make some sacrifices that will help you to get there.

Establish What You Need to Achieve and What You Need to Avoid

You cannot establish a daily routine unless you know what you want to achieve each day. On the other hand, you also need to know the bad habits you should avoid.

The first step of establishing your healthy routine, therefore, is to make two lists:

1. The things you want to achieve each day
2. The things you currently do that you want to avoid and what you could replace them with

Take a while to think about this and come back to your lists if necessary, in case you do not remember everything the first time.

Your first list must include essentials such as your job, as well as the activities needed for your health — your mealtimes, exercise periods and a good night's sleep. Do not forget to include details about your family time and leisure activities. It is essential to think of things that will enhance your well-being, rather than adding something only because it is easy to do.

Create a Daily Structure

While it is not necessary to assign an exact time for everything, it is useful to group your activities by periods of the day. It might be a good idea to have mealtimes at regular times so you can use them as landmarks. This will help you plan your activities before breakfast, before lunch, between lunch and dinner or after dinner.

Where you place activities like exercise and leisure depends entirely on yourself. Different people are at their best at different times of day, so you may for instance, wish to do your exercise before breakfast or in the early evening.

Routines such as physical structures are likely to break if they are too rigid. It is essential to build in some slack for the unexpected. For instance, if a crisis prevents you from exercising before breakfast, make sure there is an alternative substitute time for it. Make sure you build-in not only enough time to eat your healthy meals, but also to avoid walking past that vending machine, make it part of your routine to take a healthy snack with you, so you are less tempted.

Following Your Routine

At first, it is not going to be easy to remember your new routine, so you will need to be continuously reminded of it. You might find it helpful to have reminders on your phone or put fluorescent colours stickers on a wall-chart. Choose something that works well for you.

You might not get it perfectly right every day, especially at first and you should not beat yourself up about the occasional failure. However, it is worth being reasonably strict with yourself, at least initially, so that your healthy routine becomes second nature.

Following your healthy routine is the key to everything I have spoken about in this book. It is not enough just to have an understanding of healthy eating or planning exercise sessions if distractions or bad habits leave you with no time for them. Building exercise and healthy eating into your routine is the key. When you are feeling great, physically and mentally, you will wonder how you ever coped without them.

I would like to finish this book by sharing with you the quote from Jim Rohn — American author and motivational speaker. He is the man behind the famous words, "Take care of your body. It is the only place you have to live."

Life is a journey. Be happy and stay healthy. And take care of your body!

Lots of love XX

Silvana

Conclusion

Having read this book, you now have a straightforward guide on how to get fit and healthy in your own home in 20 minutes or less. As you have seen, there is no great secret about it, just applying some simple principles.

We have seen the crucial importance to your health of both a balanced diet and consistent exercise. Fad diets and pushing your exercise to the limits can actually be damaging, and even at best, they only represent unnecessary punishment for what can be achieved far more simply and enjoyably.

Many of us are motivated to diet and exercise by the desire to lose weight. This is important to your health, but measures you take to lose weight may not necessarily be healthy, whereas if you concentrate on achieving a fit, healthy, and well-balanced body, your weight will normally take care of itself.

We have seen that you do not need a fully equipped gym to get fit or an endless supply of diet food to eat healthily. I have shown you here how you can get fit and prepare healthy meals within 20 minutes in the comfort of your own home.

I have set out a simple 20-minute exercise regime you can follow without requiring any special equipment. This describes routines that allow you to warm up, exercise your upper and lower body and get the benefits of stretching.

In the same way, I have suggested easy but healthy meal ideas and a recipe book for breakfast, lunch and dinner, as well as the snacks and drinks you will need throughout the day. Instead of being based on expensive "diet foods," these meal ideas and recipes use ordinary ingredients that supply the various food groups you need, rather than the unhealthy foods we have been conditioned to reach for.

However, of course, there is no point in reading this book if you do not put its advice into practice. So what can you do now?

Firstly, you can set aside 20 minutes a day and get used to doing the exercise routine I have suggested. If you can, choose the same time each day to do your workout, so it can become a part of your daily routine. At first, you may need to force yourself, but it should quickly become a habit. Once it becomes a habit, you will love your new lifestyle.

Second, planning your meals in advance will help you to stay on track and support your healthy diet. Make sure you factor in preparation time for each meal in your busy schedule. It will take up to 20 minutes to prepare each meal I suggested in this book. Why not download my recipe book to give yourself plenty of ideas? If you have not done it yet, go to www.bit.ly/bundle-fit-and-healthy.

Of course, it is impossible to get everything into a book. If you want to know more about getting fit and healthy, you are very welcome to get in touch with me. I am inviting you to book your complimentary call with me at www.silvanahealthandnutrition.com/booking/.

Thank You

If you enjoyed this book, please consider leaving a review on the platform where you purchased it from. Even if it is only a few sentences, it would be a huge help. Your review will help this information to reach other readers, who can benefit from reading this book.

To join the mailing list for updates on future books and to receive information about health, weight loss, and nutrition, please go to www.bit.ly/silvana-signup.

About the Author

Silvana Siskov has spent many years working with her clients, helping them on the journey towards better health, weight loss and a more enjoyable life. Her passion is to encourage her clients to take action and make changes in their lives, so they can experience more happiness and a better quality of life.

Silvana understands that for many people, weight gain is just a symptom of their bad diet and unhealthy lifestyle. Through her books, she is sharing with readers her knowledge about nutrition and the experiences she has about human behaviour and our daily habits, which influence the direction of our lives.

In her first book *Get your sparkle back: 10 Steps to Weight Loss and Overcoming Emotional Eating*, Silvana looks at the struggles of emotional eaters and difficulties they face while trying to lose weight. She provides her readers with weight-loss advice and motivates them to overcome their unhealthy eating habits.

In her second book *Live Healthy on a Tight Schedule: 5 Easy Ways for Busy People to Develop Sustainable Habits Around Food, Exercise and Self-Care*, Silvana offers advice and plenty of useful tips to her readers. The guidance that Silvana gives in this book can support readers to live a healthy life, despite being very busy and having demanding jobs and a busy family life.

In Silvana's latest book *Get Fit and Healthy in Your Own Home in 20 Minutes or Less,* she is continuing to help her readers to work towards their health and weight loss goals. Following the advice given in this book, readers can benefit greatly from the meal ideas and home exercises shared in this book.

Silvana's goal is to help as many people as possible to change their unhealthy eating and lifestyle habits, so they can enjoy the benefits of good health and become fitter, slimmer and happier.

Helpful Resources

My Books:

- *Get Your Sparkle Back: 10 Steps to Weight Loss and Overcoming Emotional Eating* by Silvana Siskov, PAPERBACK ISBN: 978-1-9162424-0-1

- *Live Healthy on a Tight Schedule: 5 Easy Ways for Busy People to Develop Sustainable Habits Around Food, Exercise and Self-Care* by Silvana Siskov. PAPERBACK ISBN: 978-1-9162424-1-8

- *Get Fit and Healthy in Your Own Home in 20 Minutes or Less: An Essential Daily Exercise Plan and Simple Meal Ideas to Lose Weight and Get the Body You Want* by Silvana Siskov. PAPERBACK ISBN: 978-1-9162424-2-5

Free Mini-Courses:
- Discover 10 Secrets of Successful Weight Loss
- This Is How to Start Eating Less Sugar
- Learn How to Boost Your Energy – 11 Easy Ways

- Your Guide to a Happy and Healthy Menopause
- This Is How to Lose Weight in Your 40s and Beyond

Free Mini-Courses Available at:
www.silvanahealthandnutrition.com/course/

Book Your Complimentary Call With Me at:
www.silvanahealthandnutrition.com/booking/

Printed in Great Britain
by Amazon